INTRODUCTION TO PROTEOMICS

Introduction to Proteomics

Tools for the New Biology

By

DANIEL C. LIEBLER, PhD
College of Pharmacy
The University of Arizona
Tucson, AZ

Foreword by

JOHN R. YATES, III, PhD
Department of Cell Biology
The Scripps Research Institute
La Jolla, CA

 Humana Press
Totowa, NJ

© 2002 Humana Press Inc.
999 Riverview Drive, Suite 208
Totowa, New Jersey 07512

humanapress.com

For additional copies, pricing for bulk purchases, and/or information about other Humana titles, contact Humana at the above address or at any of the following numbers: Tel.: 973-256-1699; Fax: 973-256-8341, E-mail: humana@humanapr.com; or visit our Web
site at: www.humanapr.com

Cover design by Patricia Cleary.
Production Editor: Kim Hoather-Potter.

This publication is printed on acid-free paper.∞
ANSI Z39.48-1984 (American National Standards Institute) Permanence of Paper for Printed Library Materials.

Printed in the United States of America. 10 9 8 7 6 5 4 3

Library of Congress Cataloging-in-Publication Data

Liebler, Daniel C.
    Introduction to proteomics: tools for the new biology/Daniel C. Liebler.
    p. cm.
  Includes bibliographical references and index.
  ISBN 0-89603-991-9 (HC), ISBN 0-89603-992-7 (PB) (alk. paper)
    1. Proteins—Research—Methodology. I. Title.

QP551.L467 2002
572'.6'072—dc21   2001051465

Foreword

Mass spectrometry has evolved tremendously since Professor Klaus Biemann first analyzed amino acids in a mass spectrometer in 1958. The clear challenge in Biemann's first experiment was how to introduce nonpolar molecules into the mass spectrometer to create ions. In the years since 1958, several new ionization techniques and sample introduction methods appeared and stimulated much progress in the analysis of biomolecules. As these new ionization techniques, such as chemical ionization, field desorption, field ionization, plasma desorption, and finally fast atom bombardment (FAB) emerged, new methods for peptide and protein characterizations also developed. Mass spectrometry technology leapt forward in 1987 with the introduction of matrix-assisted laser desorption ionization (MALDI) and the application of electrospray ionization (ESI) to biomolecules. Both ionization methods led to dramatic improvements in the analysis of peptides and proteins. A key mass spectrometry technique that benefited from the new ionization methods was tandem mass spectrometry.

In the early 1980s Professor Donald Hunt began developing and applying tandem mass spectrometry to the sequence analysis of peptides and proteins. FAB, a soft ionization technique, created intact protonated molecules and allowed the refinement of approaches for peptide sequencing. FAB was a major breakthrough for peptide sequencing, because peptides could now be readily ionized without derivatization to increase volatility. By incorporating FAB with tandem mass spectrometry, a rapid peptide sequencing methodology was developed. Most approaches used off-line HPLC separations when complicated peptide mixtures were encountered. Many proteins were sequenced by this approach and many important methods were developed. Unfortunately, on-line coupling of separation methods with FAB was never able to create a robust, easy-to-use method. This problem wasn't resolved until electrospray ionization facilitated the direct coupling of separation techniques to the mass spectrometer. All aspects of peptide and protein analyses were improved by increases in the sensitivity of analysis, easier sample handling, and automation.

These developments in mass spectrometry dovetailed very nicely into the worldwide efforts to sequence the human genome. The genome sequencing efforts encompassed not only the human genome, but also genomes of many model organisms and have resulted in the generation of a large amount of sequence information. In 1993 several groups discovered that mass spectrometry data could be used to search databases to identify the protein under study. In 1994 methods to search sequence databases using tandem mass spectrometry data were developed allowing one to "look up the answer in the back of the book." If the "book" was an organism whose genome was sequenced, then the answer was most assuredly in the back. The complex issues of post-translational modifications and amino acid sequence variations can also be addressed by knowing the sequences of proteins from a genome sequence.

Interest in and use of mass spectrometry in the biological sciences has grown rapidly during the 1990s and threatens to become as ubiquitous and important as SDS-PAGE in the new millennium. Biologists will come to rely on mass spectrometry to determine the outcomes of their experiments. Given the need for biologists to use mass spectrometry technology to analyze their experiments, how does a biologist learn about the art of mass spectrometry and the methods of proteomics? This book, *Introduction to Proteomics: Tools for the New Biology* by Professor Daniel Liebler, presents a tutorial on mass spectrometry and its use in proteomics. The basics of mass spectrometers and ionization techniques are described, which is important to ascertain what type of mass spectrometer is most appropriate for a particular study. The ability to use mass spectrometry data to search databases is an important advance for the nonspecialist, because it no longer requires the development of the skills to interpret mass spectra. A basic understanding of the fundamentals of the search algorithms and their limitations is described in the book. Finally, applications of mass spectrometry to proteomics are described. This book provides an excellent introduction and overview of proteomics for the graduate student or for any biologist interested in understanding the basics of this rapidly evolving area.

John R. Yates, III
Scripps Research Institute
La Jolla, CA

Preface

This book is an introduction to the new field of proteomics. It is intended to describe how proteins and proteomes can be analyzed and studied. Despite widespread, growing interest in proteomics, an understanding of proteomics tools and technologies is only slowly penetrating the research community at large. This book addresses the need to introduce biologists to new tools and approaches, and is for both students of biology and experienced, practicing biologists. Anyone who has taken a graduate level biochemistry course should be able to take from this book a reasonable understanding of what proteomics is all about and how it is practiced. The experienced biologist should encounter much here that is familiar, but refocused to facilitate studies of the proteome.

The achievement of long-sought milestones in genome sequencing, analytical instrumentation, computing power, and user-friendly software tools has irrevocably changed the practice of biology. After years of studying the individual components of living systems, we can now study the systems themselves in comprehensive scope and in exquisite molecular detail. We therefore face the tasks of effectively employing new technologies, of dealing with mountains of data, and, most important, of adjusting our thinking to understand complex systems as opposed to their individual components.

Introduction to Proteomics: Tools for the New Biology had its origins in a short course on peptide sequencing by mass spectrometry, which was taught by Dr. Donald F. Hunt at the 1998 Association of Biomedical Resource Facilities meeting in Durham, North Carolina. At that time, my colleague Dr. Tom McClure and I were establishing a new proteomics facility in the Center for Toxicology and the Arizona Cancer Center at the University of Arizona. Tom attended the Hunt course and, upon his return, taught the material to a handful of us. We subsequently put together a four-day workshop on mass spectrometry and proteomics, which we taught to 50 participants at the University of Arizona in August, 1999. The participants included graduate students, laboratory staff, and faculty. The enthusiastic response to this workshop reflected the need for some accessible means of introducing scientists to the new techniques of proteomics and their potential applications in research. That experience provided the impetus for this book.

This is a book for beginners. My goal here is to familiarize the inexperienced reader with the important tools and applications of proteomics. Thus the description of certain instrumentation and applications is not highly rigorous. This book is not intended to be a laboratory manual or a compilation of the latest techniques. There are several excellent volumes available that provide more detailed descriptions of protein analytical techniques, mass spectrometry instrumentation and techniques, and applications of these technologies. The evolution of methods and applications in this area is now so rapid that no book really could be truly up-to-date. What is exciting about my experience in introducing proteomics to colleagues has been the creativity with which they then apply these tools. Ultimately, the exciting potential of proteomics rests with those who can put new technologies to work to address important questions.

I have divided the book into three parts. Part I introduces the subject of proteomics, describes its place in the new biology, and examines the nature of proteomes. Part II introduces the tools of proteomics research and explains how they work. Part III explains how these tools are integrated to solve different types of problems in biology.

I would like to thank Jeanne Burr, Laura Tiscareno, Julie Jones, Dan Mason, Beau Hansen, Hamid Badghisi, Linda Manza, Richard Vaillancourt, Tom McClure, Arpad Somogyi, and George Tsaprailis, who provided valuable suggestions, read and commented on several drafts of book chapters and provided sample data for some of the illustrations. I thank Elizabeth Hedger for excellent secretarial assistance. Finally, I thank my wife Karen and my son Andrew for their patience with me every time I went off with my laptop to write.

Daniel C. Liebler, PhD

Contents

I Proteomics and the Proteome

1 Proteomics and the New Biology

1.1. The New Biology

Proteomics is the study of the proteome, the protein complement of the genome. The terms "proteomics" and "proteome" were coined by Marc Wilkins and colleagues in the early 1990s and mirror the terms "genomics" and "genome," which describe the entire collection of genes in an organism. These "-omics" terms symbolize a redefinition of how we think about biology and the workings of living systems (**Fig. 1**). Until the mid-1990s, biochemists, molecular biologists, and cell biologists studied individual genes and proteins or small clusters of related components of specific biochemical pathways. The techniques then available—Northern blots (for gene expression) and Western blots (for protein levels)—made charting the status of more than a handful of genes or proteins a formidable analytical task.

Three developments changed the biological landscape and formed the foundation of the new biology. The first was the growth of gene, expressed sequence tag (EST), and protein-sequence databases during the 1990s. These resources became ever more useful as partial catalogs of expressed genes in many organisms. The genome-sequencing projects of the late 1990s yielded complete genomic sequences of bacteria, yeast, nematodes, and drosophila and culminated recently in the complete sequence of the human genome. Sequences of plant genomes and those of other widely studied animals also are recently completed or are approaching completion. These genome-sequence

From: *Introduction to Proteomics: Tools for the New Biology*
By: D. C. Liebler © Humana Press, Inc., Totowa, NJ

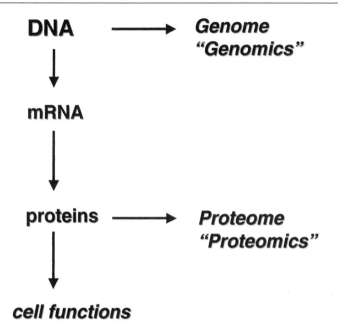

Fig. 1. Biochemical context of genomics and proteomics.

databases are the catalogs from which much of our understanding of living systems eventually will be extracted.

The second key development is the introduction of user-friendly, browser-based bioinformatics tools to extract information from these databases. It is now possible to search entire genomes for specific nucleic acid or protein sequences in seconds. Such database search tools are integrated with other tools and databases to predict the functions of the protein products based on the occurrence of specific functional domains or motifs. This array of free web-based tools now enables the biologist to probe structures and functions of genes and gene products and to explore a great deal of interesting biochemistry right from a desktop computer.

The third key development is the oligonucleotide microarray. The array contains a series of gene-specific oligonucleotides or cDNA sequences on a slide or a chip. By applying a mixture of fluorescently labeled DNAs from a sample of interest to the array, one can probe

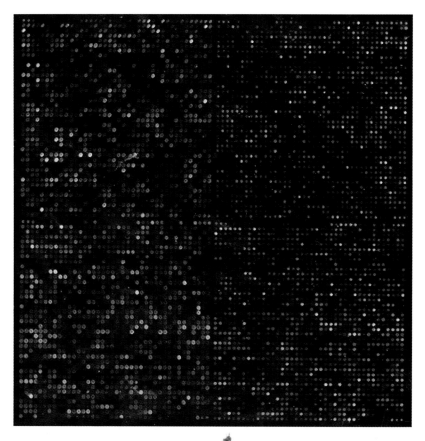

Fig. 2. The yeast genome on a chip. This yeast cDNA microarray was produced by the laboratory of Dr. Patrick Brown at Stanford University (http://cmgm.stanford.edu/pbrown/).

the expression of thousands of genes at once. One array can replace thousands of Northern-blot analyses and can be done in the time it would take to do one Northern. Moreover, with two-color fluorescent probe labeling, expression of genes in two different samples can be compared directly on one slide or chip.

An array slide containing unique sequences for each of the 6000 genes in the *Sacchromyces cerevisiea* genome is pictured in **Fig. 2**. From this single array, one can assess the expression of all genes in the yeast genome. Such pictures vividly confront us with the greatest challenge of the new biology. *We can see the whole system*, but the information contained in these thousands of data points is beyond our ability to interpret intuitively. New clustering algorithms, self-organizing maps, and similar tools represent the latest approaches to rendering the data in ways that biologists can comprehend.

The most important thing about arrays in this context is that they have challenged biologists to think *big*. A cell has thousands or tens of thousands of genes that may be expressed in varying combinations. The life and death of cells is dictated by the expression of these genes and the activities of their protein products. Each protein, whether a transmembrane receptor, a transcription factor, a protein kinase, or a chaperone, expresses a function that assumes significance only in the context of all the other functions and activities also being expressed in the same cell. Thus, biologists are now struggling to think big, to understand systems rather than just components, and to make sense of complexity.

1.2. Proteomics? That's Just What We Used to Call Protein Chemistry!

A common response to new ideas, terms, and approaches is to claim that they are not really new after all. For this reason, it is important to explain just what are the differences between proteomics and protein biochemistry. Both proteomics and protein chemistry involve protein identification, so what's the difference? **Table 1** provides a short summary of the key features to consider. Protein chemistry involves the study of protein structure and function and is most commonly manifest in the fields of physical biochemistry or mechanistic enzymology. The work generally involves complete sequence analysis, structure determination, and modeling studies to explore how structure governs function. Physical biochemists and enzymologists typically study one protein or multisubunit protein complex at a time.

Proteomics is the study of multiprotein systems, in which the focus is on the interplay of multiple, distinct proteins in their roles as part of a larger system or network. Analyses are directed at complex mixtures and identification is not by complete sequence analysis,

Table 1
Differences Between Protein Chemistry and Proteomics

Protein chemistry	Proteomics
• Individual proteins	• Complex mixtures
• Complete sequence analysis	• Partial sequence analysis
• Emphasis on structure and function	• Emphasis on identification by database matching
• Structural biology	• Systems biology

but instead by partial sequence analysis with the aid of database matching tools. The context of proteomics is systems biology, rather than structural biology. In other words, the point of proteomics is to characterize the behavior of the system rather than the behavior of any single component.

1.3. If We Can Measure Gene Expression, Why Bother With Proteomics?

Gene microarrays offer a snapshot of the expression of many or all genes in a cell. Unfortunately, the levels of mRNAs do not necessarily predict the levels of the corresponding proteins in a cell. Differing stability of mRNAs and different efficiencies in translation can affect the generation of new proteins. Once formed, proteins differ significantly in stability and turnover rates. Many proteins involved in signal transduction, transcription-factor regulation, and cell-cycle control are rapidly turned over as a means of regulating their activities. Finally, mRNA levels tell us nothing about the regulatory status of the corresponding proteins, whose activities and functions are subject to many endogenous posttranslational modifications and other modifications by environmental agents.

1.4. Proteomics: An Analytical Challenge

The problem of how to measure the expression of many or all of the genes in an organism simultaneously seems to have been solved by the introduction of cDNA or oligonucleotide microarrays. Analysis of gene expression by microarrays and related methods relies on two essential tools, polymerase chain reaction (PCR) and hybridization of oligonucleotides to complementary sequences. Unfortunately, there are no analogous tools available for protein analysis. First, there is no protein equivalent of PCR. It is not currently possible to induce polypeptide molecules to replicate themselves in a manner analogous to oligonucleotide replication through PCR. Whereas a small amount of oligonucleotide can be amplified through PCR, a small amount of a polypeptide must be detected and analyzed without any amplification.

Second, proteins do not specifically hybridize to complementary amino acid sequences. Watson-Crick base-pairing allows oligonucleotides to hybridize to complementary sequences. A defined complementary oligonucleotide sequence can serve as a highly specific probe to which a specific mRNA or other nucleic acid fragment can bind. This specificity allows a particular spot on the microarray to recognize a unique sequence. Although antibodies and oligonucleotide aptamers can recognize specific peptides or proteins, recognition cannot be predicted simply on the basis of sequence, as it can for oligonucleotides.

Another problem peculiar to proteomics is that each protein gene product does not necessarily give rise to only one molecular entity in the cell. This is because proteins are posttranslationally modified. The extent and variety of modification varies with individual proteins, regulatory mechanisms within the cell, and environmental factors. Consequently, many proteins are present in multiple forms. The necessity of detecting and differentiating between multiple protein products of any particular gene adds much to the analytical challenge of proteomics.

Analysis of the proteome thus requires a different set of tools than does gene-expression analysis. The task of characterizing the proteome requires analytical methods to detect and quantify proteins in their modified and unmodified forms. How we deal with this task is the subject of this book.

1.5. Tools of Proteomics

Despite the relative disadvantages of analytical proteomics described earlier, the task of characterizing the proteome and its components is now practically achievable. This is because the development and integration of four important tools provide investigators with sensitive, specific means of identifying and characterizing proteins.

The first tool is the database. Protein, EST, and complete genome-sequence databases collectively provide a complete catalog of all proteins expressed in organisms for which the databases are available. Based on analyses of all the coding sequences for *Drosophila*, for example, we know that there are 110 *Drosophila* genes that code for proteins with EGF-like domains and 87 genes that code for proteins with tyrosine kinase catalytic domains. Accordingly, when doing proteomics in *Drosophila*, we are searching a large, but *known* index of possible proteins. When searched with limited sequence information or even raw mass spectral data (*see* below), we can identify a protein component from a match with a database entry.

The second tool is mass spectrometry (MS). MS instrumentation has undergone tremendous change over the past decade, culminating in the development of highly sensitive, robust instruments that can reliably analyze biomolecules, particularly proteins and peptides. MS instrumentation can offer three types of analyses, all of which are highly useful in proteomics. First, MS can provide accurate molecular mass measurements of intact proteins as large as 100 kDa or more. Thus, MS analysis, rather that migration on sodium dodecyl sulfate-polyacrylamide gel electrophoresis (SDS-PAGE) is the best way to estimate protein masses. Highly accurate protein mass measurements generally are of limited utility, however, because they often are not sufficiently sensitive and because net mass often is insufficient for unambiguous protein identification. MS also can provide accurate mass measurements of peptides from proteolytic digests. In contrast to whole protein mass measurements, peptide mass measurements can be done with higher sensitivity and mass accuracy. The data from these peptide mass measurements can be searched directly against databases, frequently to obtain definitive identification of the target proteins. Finally, MS analyses can provide sequence analysis of peptides obtained from proteolytic digests. Indeed, MS is now considered the state-of-the-art in peptide-sequence analysis. MS sequence data provide the most powerful and unambiguous approach to protein identification.

The third essential tool for proteomics is an emerging collection of software that can match MS data with specific protein sequences in databases. As noted earlier, it is possible to determine the sequence of a peptide from MS data. However, this *de novo* sequence interpretation is a relatively laborious task, particularly when one has to interpret hundreds or thousands of spectra. These software tools take *uninterpreted* MS data and match it to sequences in protein, EST, and genome-sequence databases with the aid of specialized algorithms. The most useful aspect of these tools is that they permit the automated survey of large amounts of MS data for protein-sequence matches. The investigator then can inspect the results and evaluate the quality of the data in far less time than it would take to interpret each spectrum manually.

The fourth essential tool in proteomics is analytical protein-separation technology. Protein separations serve two purposes in proteomics. First, they simplify complex protein mixtures by resolving them into individual proteins or small groups of proteins. Second, because they also permit apparent differences in protein levels to be compared between two samples, protein analytical separations allow investigators to target specific proteins for analysis. Certainly, two-dimensional SDS-PAGE (2D-SDS-PAGE) is most widely associated with proteomics. Two-dimensional gels represent perhaps the best single technique for resolving proteins in a complex sample. However, other protein-separation techniques, including 1D-SDS-PAGE, high-performance liquid chromatography (HPLC), capillary electrophoresis (CE), isoelectric focusing (IEF), and affinity chromatography all can be useful tools in analytical proteomics. Perhaps most powerful is the integration of different protein and peptide separations as multidimensional techniques. For example, ion-exchange liquid chromatography (LC) in tandem with reverse-phase (RP)-HPLC is a powerful tool for resolving complex peptide mixtures.

It is the integration of these four tools that provides the current technology of proteomics. Each of these capabilities is rapidly evolving from a technical standpoint. We will consider each of these sets of analytical tools in subsequent chapters in this book.

1.6. Applications of Proteomics

Proteomics technology is indeed impressive, but what does characterizing the proteome amount to in practical terms? In current practice, proteomics encompasses four principal applications. These are: 1) mining, 2) protein-expression profiling, 3) protein-network mapping, and 4) mapping of protein modifications. These each will be defined briefly below and in detail in subsequent chapters in this book.

Mining is simply the exercise of identifying all (or as many as possible) of the proteins in a sample. The point of mining is to catalog the proteome directly, rather than to infer the composition of the proteome from expression data for genes (e.g., by microarrays). Mining is the ultimate brute-force exercise in proteomics: one simply resolves proteins to the greatest extent possible and then uses MS and associated database and software tools to identify what is found. There are several approaches to mining and each offers advantages. What these approaches collectively offer is the ability to confirm by direct analysis what could only be inferred from gene-expression data.

Protein-expression profiling is the identification of proteins in a particular sample as a function of a particular state of the organism or cell (e.g., differentiation, developmental state, or disease state) or as a function of exposure to a drug, chemical, or physical stimulus. Expression profiling is actually a specialized form of mining. It is most commonly practiced as a differential analysis, in which two states of a particular system are compared. For example, normal and diseased cells or tissues can be compared to determine which proteins are expressed differently in one state compared to the other. This information has tremendous appeal as a means of detecting potential targets for drug therapy in disease.

Protein-network mapping is the proteomics approach to determining how proteins interact with each other in living systems. Most proteins carry out their functions in close association with other proteins. It is these interactions that determine the functions of protein functional networks, such as signal-transduction cascades and complex biosynthetic or degradation pathways. Much has been learned about protein-protein interactions through in vitro studies with individual, purified proteins and with the yeast two-hybrid system. However, proteomics approaches offer the opportunity to characterize more complex networks through the creative pairing of affinity-capture techniques coupled with analytical proteomics methods. Proteomics approaches have been used to identify components of multiprotein complexes. Multiple complexes are involved in point-to-point signal-transduction pathways in cells. Protein-network profiling would offer the ability to assess at once the status of all the participants in the pathway. As such, protein-network profiling represents one of the most ambitious and potentially powerful future applications of proteomics.

Mapping of protein modifications is the task of identifying how and where proteins are modified. Many common posttranslational modifications govern the targeting, structure, function, and turnover of proteins. In addition, many environmental chemicals, drugs, and endogenous chemicals give rise to reactive electrophiles that modify proteins. A variety of analytical tools have been developed to identify modified proteins and the nature of the modifications. Modified proteins can be detected with antibodies (e.g., for specific phosphorylated amino acid residues), but the precise sequence sites of a specific modification often are not known. Proteomics approaches offer the best means of establishing both the nature and sequence specificity of posttranslational modifications. The extension of this approach to simultaneous characterization of the modification status of regulated proteins in a network again represents a powerful extension of proteomics technology. These approaches will provide fresh avenues of approach to questions of how chemical modification of the proteome affects living systems.

Suggested Reading

Brown, P. O. and Botstein, D. (1999) Exploring the new world of the genome with DNA microarrays. *Nat. Genet.* **21,** 33–37.

DeRisi, J. L., Iyer, V. R., and Brown, P. O. (1997) Exploring the metabolic and genetic control of gene expression on a genomic scale. *Science* **278,** 680–686.

Eisen, M. B., Spellman, P. T., Brown, P. O., and Botstein, D. (1998) Cluster analysis and display of genome-wide expression patterns. *Proc. Natl. Acad. Sci. USA* **95,** 14,863–14,868.

Fields, S. (2001) Proteomics. Proteomics in genomeland. *Science* **291,** 1221–1224.

Lander, E. S., Linton, L. M., Birren, B., Nusbaum, C., et al. (2001) Initial sequencing and analysis of the human genome. *Nature* **409,** 860–921.

Lashkari, D. A., DeRisi, J. L., McCusker, J. H., Namath, A. F., Gentile, C., Hwang, S. Y., et al. (1997) Yeast microarrays for genome wide parallel genetic and gene expression analysis. *Proc. Natl. Acad. Sci. USA* **94,** 13,057–13,062.

Pandey, A. and Mann, M. (2000) Proteomics to study genes and genomes. *Nature* **405,** 837–846.

Venter, J. C., Adams, M. D., Myers, E. W., Li, P. W., Mural, R. J., et al. (2001) The sequence of the human genome. *Science* **291,** 1304–1351.

Wilkins, M. R., Sanchez, J. C., Gooley, A. A., Appel, R. D., Humphery-Smith, I., Hochstrasser, D. F., and Williams, K. L. (1996) Progress with proteome projects: why all proteins expressed by a genome should be identified and how to do it. *Biotechnol. Genet. Eng. Rev.* **13,** 19–50.

2 The Proteome

2.1. The Proteome and the Genome

Each of our cells contains all the information necessary to make a complete human being. However, not all the genes are expressed in all the cells. Genes that code for enzymes essential to basic cellular functions (e.g., glucose catabolism, DNA synthesis) are expressed in virtually all cells, whereas those with highly specialized functions are expressed only in specific cell types (e.g., rhodopsin in retinal pigment epithelium). Thus, all cells express: 1) genes whose protein products provide essential functions, and 2) genes whose protein products provide unique cell-specific functions. Thus, every organism has one genome, but many proteomes.

The proteome in any cell thus represents some subset of all possible gene products. However, this does not mean that the proteome is simpler than the genome. In fact, the opposite is certainly true. Any protein, though a product of a single gene, may exist in multiple forms that vary within a particular cell or between different cells. Indeed, most proteins exist in several modified forms. These modifications affect protein structure, localization, function, and turnover.

In this chapter, we look at the proteome in five different ways. First, we briefly consider the "life-cycle" of proteins—from their appearance as translation products in ribosomes to their many modifications and their ultimate degradation. Second, we consider proteins as modular structures that can be classified in groups based on sequence motifs, domain structures, and biochemical functions. Third, we consider the distribution of the genome into functional families of proteins.

From: *Introduction to Proteomics: Tools for the New Biology*
By: D. C. Liebler © Humana Press, Inc., Totowa, NJ

Fourth, we look at the proteome through genomic sequences, which indicate the diversity and redundancy of functions in living systems. Finally, we consider the factors that dictate how much of any protein is present in a cell at any one time, and how that influences the difficulty of finding it by analytical proteomics methods.

2.2. The Life and Death of a Protein

Proteins are synthesized by the translation of mRNAs into polypeptides on ribosomes. In most cases, the initial polypeptide-translation product undergoes some type of modification before it assumes its functional role in a living system. These changes are broadly termed "posttranslational modifications" and encompass a wide variety of reversible and irreversible chemical reactions. Approximately 200 different types of posttranslational modifications have been reported. Some of these are summarized in **Fig. 1**, which depicts the life cycle of a prototypical protein.

The protein is born as a ribosomal translation product of an mRNA sequence. Folding and oxidation of cysteine thiols to disulfides confers secondary structure on the random-coil polypeptide. A number of "permanent" modifications, such as carboxylation of glutamate residues or removal of the N-terminal methionine, can occur early in the life of the polypeptide. Further processing in the Golgi apparatus often results in glycosylation. Specific delivery of the protein to specific subcellular or extracellular compartments is often achieved with leader or signal sequences, which may be proteolytically cleaved. Prosthetic groups may be added. Combination with other proteins forms multisubunit complexes. Palmitoylation or prenylation of cysteine residues assists anchoring of proteins in or on membranes. These more or less "permanent" modifications and transport ultimately result in the delivery of functional proteins to specific locations in cells.

At their cellular destinations, proteins carry out their many functions. The activities of many proteins are then controlled by posttranslational modifications. The most prominent and best-understood of these is phosphorylation of serine, threonine, or tyrosine residues. Phosphorylation may activate or inactivate enzymes, alter protein-protein interactions and associations, change protein structures, and target proteins for degradation. Protein phosphorylation regulates protein function in diverse contexts and appears to be a key switch

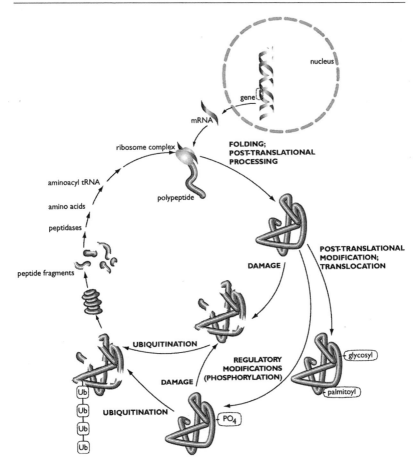

Fig. 1. The life cycle of a protein.

for rapid on-off control of signaling cascades, cell-cycle control, and other key cellular functions.

Proteins also are subject to wear and tear. The ubiquitous presence of free radicals and other oxidants in biological systems leads to oxidative protein damage. Several amino acids are susceptible to oxidation, particularly cysteine thiols. Methionine, tryptophan, histidine, and tyrosine residues also are easily oxidized. Proteins also are subject to attack by products of lipid and carbohydrate oxidation, including reactive α,β-unsaturated carbonyl compounds. In addition to these endogenous sources of protein modification, environmental agents, including radiation, chemicals, and drugs can covalently or oxidatively modify proteins. Many of these modifications can inactivate proteins, but virtually all produce some modifications of protein structure.

Protein modifications appear to be critical to initiating processes that ultimately degrade proteins. Phosphorylation of some proteins is rapidly followed by conjugation with ubiquitin, which leads to degradation by the 26S proteasomal complex. There evidently are other stimuli for protein ubiquitination and turnover, including oxidative damage and other protein modifications. Proteins also undergo degradation by lysosomal enzymes.

The foregoing sketch of the life of a protein illustrates a key point about the proteome. Any protein may be present in many forms at any one time in a cell. Collectively, the proteome of a cell comprises all of these many forms of all expressed proteins. This certainly makes the proteome bewilderingly complex. On the other hand, the status of the proteome reflects the state of the cell in all its functions.

2.3. Proteins as Modular Structures

Another way to look at proteins is to think of them as modular or mosaic structures. Certain amino acid sequences tend to form secondary structures, such as α-helices, β-sheets, or random-coil structures. However, specific amino acid sequences and secondary structures derived from these sequences also confer unique properties and functions. In this way, segments of amino acid sequences can be considered as functional building blocks or modules. From these modules, Nature has assembled a tool box from which to build proteins with diverse, yet related functions.

The modular units in proteins that confer specific properties and functions are referred to as "motifs" or "domains". These are recognizable sequences that confer similar properties or functions when they occur in a variety of proteins. In common usage these terms often overlap. In some cases, amino acid sequences within motifs and domains are highly conserved and do not vary from protein to protein. In other cases, some key amino acids occur in a reproducible relationship to each other in a sequence, even though various substitutions in other amino acids occur.

Even some short sequences can confer specificity for certain modifications. For example, proteins that undergo N-glycosylation tend to display a tripeptide sequence "Asn-Xaa-Ser/Thr," in which the target asparagine is followed by any amino acid and then either a serine or threonine residue. If the "Xaa" is a proline, glycosylation is blocked. Although this sequence does not ensure N-glycosylation, it does provide a signature motif that can offer clues to possible biochemical roles.

Longer amino acid sequences often form domains, which confer specific properties or functions on a protein. Some domain structures simply refer simply to sequences that confer a bulk physical property to a segment of the polypeptide, such as transmembrane domains, which simply form helices that span a lipid bilayer membrane. Other domain structures provide hydrogen bonding or other contacts for key enzyme substrates or prosthetic groups. For example, eukaryotic serine/threonine kinases display a core domain that includes a glycine-rich region surrounding a lysine residue involved in ATP binding and a conserved aspartate residue that functions as a catalytic center. In many cases, domains are made up of combinations of units of secondary structure, such as helix-loop-helix domains.

The significance of motifs and domains for proteomics is that they represent the translation of peptide sequence to protein functions. In cases where domains and motifs confer known properties or functions, their occurrence in proteins of unknown function offer hints as to their cellular roles. In short, analytical proteomics can define sequence and sequence can define biological function.

2.4. Functional Protein Families

Another way to look at the proteome is to divide it into families of proteins that carry out related functions. For example, some proteins serve structural roles, some are participants in signaling pathways, and others handle essential metabolic chores such as nucleic acid synthesis or carbohydrate catabolism. Based on classification by domain content and associated functional roles, Venter and colleagues (2001) estimated the division of protein functions in proteins encoded by the human genome (**Fig. 2**).

Enzymes involved in intermediary metabolism and nucleic acid metabolism account for about 15% of the proteins represented in the proteome. Proteins associated with structure and protein synthesis

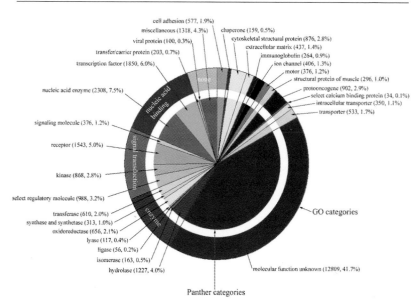

Fig. 2. Functions assigned to predicted protein products of human genes. (Reprinted with permission from Venter et al. (2001) *Science* **291**: 1304–1351. Copyright 2001, American Association for the Advancement of Science.)

and turnover (cytoskeletal proteins, ribosomal proteins, chaperones, and mediators of protein degradation) account collectively for another 15–20%. Another 20–25% consists of signaling proteins and DNA binding proteins. Although these numbers offer a useful perspective on how the genome is divided by protein functions, they do not tell us how much of any protein or protein class is expressed at any given time in a cell. Approximately 40% of the genome encodes protein products with no known function. Assigning functions to these gene products represents the most fundamental challenge for human functional genomics.

2.5. Deducing the Proteome from the Genome

One of the most interesting questions facing researchers who characterize genomes in an organism is "How many genes are there?" The answer to this question can give us some idea of how many

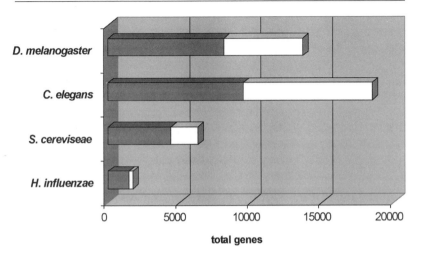

Fig. 3. Predicted protein products of genes from *H. influenzae* (1,709 genes), *S. cerevisiae* (6,241 genes), *C. elegans* (18,424 genes), and *D. melanogaster* (13,601 genes). The dark bar segments depict genes coding for unique proteins; the light bar segments depict genes coding for paralogs. (Adapted with permission from Rubin et al. (2000) *Science* **287:** 2204–2215. Copyright 2000, American Association for the Advancement of Science.)

proteins may exist in the proteome. Complete genomic sequences of several organisms have been completed and these data have allowed analysts to predict the products of all the organism's genes. Moreover, based on the predicted amino acid sequences of each gene product, these proteins have been classified on the basis of the domains and sequence motifs they contain. For example, 119 of the genes of the *Saccharomyces cerevisiae* genome encode proteins with eukaryotic protein kinase domains, whereas 47 others encode proteins with C2H2-type zinc-finger domains. Comparisons of domain-sequence characteristics with genomic sequences reveals many other protein types encoded in an organism's genome.

Recent analyses of the *S. cerevisiae, Caenorhabditis elegans*, and *Drosophila* genomes have revealed very interesting relationships between the size of the genomes and the predicted content of the proteomes for these organisms. Gerald Rubin and colleagues have classified the predicted protein products of the *H. influenzae*, *S. cerevisiae*, *C. elegans*, and *Drosophila* genomes based on the presence of specific domains (**Fig. 3**). Comparison of all the predicted protein products indicated the occurrence of proteins whose sequence differed only slightly from others in the genome. Correction for these redundant protein products, termed "paralogs," allowed the calculation of a "core proteome" for each organism. This core proteome represents the basic collection of distinct protein families for an organism.

A look at the the core proteomes for these organisms illustrates two interesting aspects of the proteome. First, the relationship between the complexity of an organism and the number of genes in its genome is not simple. Certainly, the yeast has more genes than the bacterium, yet fewer than the worm and the fly. However, the fly (*Drosophila melanogaster*) is a much more complicated organism than the worm (*C. elegans*), yet it has fewer genes (13,601 vs 18,424 in the worm) and a smaller core proteome (8065 distinct proteins vs 9543 in the fly). This suggests that biological complexity does not come simply from greater numbers of genes. Instead, more complex regulation of the genes and the functions of the protein products may account for the greater complexity of the fly.

Second, the number of paralogs increases dramatically in the worm and the fly. This reflects the fact that about half of the genes in the worm and the fly are near-duplicates of other genes. These duplicate-containing gene families often appear as gene clusters on the same chromosome.

The recent completion of the human genome sequence has provided evidence that the human genome encodes between 30,000 and 40,000 genes. In view of the tremendous difference in complexity of the human organism compared to the worm, it is indeed surprising that the human genome encodes only about twice as many genes as that of the worm. Reliable estimates of the numbers of unique genes vs paralogs are not yet available. Nevertheless, it is already becoming axiomatic that the complexity of the human organism lies in the diversity of human proteomes, rather than in the size of the human genome.

2.6. Gene Expression, Codon Bias, and Protein Levels

One of the key issues encountered by investigators who study the proteome is how much of a particular protein is expressed in a cell.

Expression levels of proteins vary tremendously, from a few copies to more than a million. It is important to realize in this context that the level of a protein expressed in a cell has little to do with its significance. Essential enzymes of intermediary metabolism or structural proteins often are present at levels in the thousands of copies per cell or more, whereas certain protein kinases involved in cell-cycle regulation are found at only tens of copies per cell. *S. cerevisiae* contains approx 6000 genes, of which about 4000 are expressed at any given time, based on measurements of mRNA levels.

The level of any protein in a cell at any given time is controlled by: 1) the rate of transcription of the gene, 2) the efficiency of translation of mRNA into protein, and 3) the rate of degradation of the protein in the cell. Gene expression certainly can dictate protein levels to a considerable extent. However, a number of studies indicate that gene expression *per se* does not really correlate that well with protein levels. This finding certainly reflects the influences of the other two factors mentioned earlier. It also is an important reminder of the limitations of gene-expression analyses (such as microarrays).

Many genes are regulated by inducible transcription factors, which are regulated in turn by a wide variety of environmental influences. However, an intrinsic determinant of the level of expression of many genes is a phenomenon referred to as "codon bias." This term describes the tendency of an organism to prefer certain codons over others that code for the same amino acid in the gene sequence. Thus, genes containing codon variants that are less preferred tend to be expressed at a lower level. Calculated codon bias values for yeast genes range from approx –0.2 to 1.0, where a value of 1.0 favors the highest level of gene expression. Most yeast genes display codon bias values of less than 0.25 and are expected to be expressed at relatively low levels.

Studies in yeast have compared protein levels, mRNA expression, and codon bias for a number of proteins. While there is some disagreement as to the particulars, the following generalizations can be drawn.

- Genes with low codon bias values tend to be expressed at low levels, whether analyzed on the basis of mRNA expression or protein levels.
- mRNA levels correlate poorly ($r < 0.4$) with protein levels when genes with codon bias values of 0.25 or less (i.e., most genes)

are considered. However, the correlation between mRNA levels and protein levels is much higher ($r > 0.85$) for the most highly expressed genes (i.e., those with codon bias values above 0.5).

- Longer-lived proteins appear to be present in higher abundance than short-lived proteins (i.e., those proteins that are degraded rapidly).

Thus, although gene-expression measurements may indicate changes in protein levels, it is difficult to infer protein expression from gene expression.

2.7. Conclusion and Significance for Analytical Proteomics

The proteome in essentially any organism is a collection of somewhere between 30 and 80% of the possible gene products. Most of these proteins are expressed at relatively low levels (10^1–10^2 per cell), although some are expressed at much higher levels (10^4–10^6 per cell). Regardless of the absolute level of expression of the polypeptide gene products, most proteins exist in multiple posttranslationally modified forms. This situation poses the greatest challenge for proteomic analysis: we must find ways to detect a large number of distinct molecular species, most of which are present at relatively low levels and many of which exist in multiple modified forms. The next section of the book describes the tools we can bring to bear on this daunting analytical problem.

Suggested Reading

Apweiler, R., Attwood, T. K., Bairoch, A., Bateman, A., Birney, E., et al. (2001) The InterPro database, an integrated documentation resource for protein families, domains and functional sites. *Nucleic Acids Res.* **29,** 37–40.

Coghlan, A. and Wolfe, K. H. (2000) Relationship of codon bias to mRNA concentration and protein length in Saccharomyces cerevisiae. *Yeast* **16,** 1131–1145.

Gygi, S. P., Rochon, Y., Franza, B. R., and Aebersold, R. (1999) Correlation between protein and mRNA abundance in yeast. *Mol. Cell Biol.* **19,** 1720–1730.

Rubin, G. M., Yandell, M. D., Wortman, J. R., Gabor Miklos, G. L., Nelson, C. R., et al. (2000) Comparative genomics of the eukaryotes. *Science* **287,** 2204–2215.

Venter, J. C., Adams, M. D., Myers, E. W., Li, P. W., Mural, R. J., et al. (2001) The sequence of the human genome. *Science* **291,** 1304–1351.

II Tools of Proteomics

3 Overview of Analytical Proteomics

Before we consider the elements of analytical proteomics in detail, let's sketch out the basic approach. Analytical protein identification is built around one essential fact: most peptide sequences of approximately six or more amino acids are largely unique in the proteome of an organism. Put another way, a typical six amino acid peptide maps to a single gene product. Thus, if we can obtain the sequence of the peptide or if we can accurately measure its mass, we can identify the protein it came from simply by finding its match in a database of protein sequences (**Fig. 1**). Of course, some hexapeptides may map to more than one protein, but multiple "hits" typically come from highly conserved regions of related proteins (such as the paralogs discussed in Chapter 2). If one can obtain sequences of several peptides that map to the same gene product, this strengthens the validity of the match. Accordingly, the essence of analytical proteomics is to convert proteins to peptides, obtain sequences of the peptides, and then identify the corresponding proteins from matching sequences in a database.

Figure 1 depicts the essential elements of the analytical proteomics approach. Most analytical proteomics problems begin with a protein mixture. This mixture contains intact proteins of varying molecular weights, modifications, and solubilities. Before peptide sequences can be obtained, the proteins must be cleaved to peptides. This is because the mass spectrometers used to measure peptide masses or obtain peptide sequences cannot perform these measurements

From: *Introduction to Proteomics: Tools for the New Biology*
By: D. C. Liebler © Humana Press, Inc., Totowa, NJ

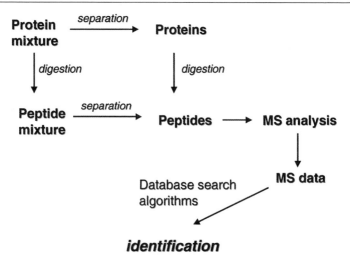

Fig. 1. General flow scheme for proteomic analysis.

directly on intact proteins. Although modern MS instruments can obtain a tremendous amount of data even from relatively complex peptide mixtures, simplification of the mixtures allows data to be collected on the greatest number of components.

Thus, to analyze protein mixtures by MS, the highly complex mixture of many components must be separated into somewhat less complex mixtures containing fewer components. It is possible to separate the intact proteins first and then cleave them into peptides. However, it is also possible to cleave the proteins into peptides first and then separate the peptides prior to analysis. The resolution of proteins and peptides and the cleavage of proteins to peptides are described in Chapters 4 and 5.

The peptides are then analyzed by either of two types of mass spectrometers. The first type, referred to as Matrix Assisted Laser Desorption Ionization-Time of Flight (MALDI-TOF) instruments, are used primarily to measure the masses of peptides. The second type, referred to as Electrospray Ionization (ESI)-tandem MS instruments, are used to obtain sequence data for peptides. These instruments are described in Chapter 6.

The data from the mass spectrometers is then used, with the aid of specialized software, to identify peptides and peptide sequences from databases that match the data from the analyses. This essentially establishes the identity of the proteins in the original mixture. This type of matching is done without directly interpreting peptide sequences from the MS data. The use of these software tools and protein-identification approaches is described in Chapters 7–9.

That's basically it. Analytical proteomics is essentially one assay, in which protein mixtures are converted to peptide mixtures, peptide MS data are obtained, and the corresponding proteins are identified by software-assisted database searching. What makes proteomics so powerful is that this one assay can be applied to many different protein samples generated from a variety of experimental designs. What makes proteomics so versatile is the great variety of "front-end" experiments that can be done to obtain the samples to be analyzed by this one assay. These front-end experiments and their applications are the subject of the third part of this book.

4 Analytical Protein and Peptide Separations

4.1. Overview

This chapter describes the approaches used to prepare protein samples for MS analysis. At this stage of proteomic analysis, we must do two things (**Fig. 1**). First, we must convert proteins to peptides. This is generally done with proteolytic enzymes. Second, we must separate very complex mixtures of proteins or peptides into somewhat less complex mixtures. This gives the MS instruments a better opportunity to obtain useful data on the components of the mixture. There is no obligatory order for these two steps. We can first separate proteins, then digest them and analyze the peptides. Alternatively, we can first digest a complex mixture of proteins to peptides, and then resolve the peptides. Each approach has advantages and drawbacks, which will be discussed here.

4.2. Complex Protein and Peptide Mixtures

Before we get into the approaches to separation and digestion, let's consider why the problem of complex protein mixtures is an issue. The MS instruments used to obtain data on peptides are capable of extracting a great deal of information from relatively complex mixtures. However, our chances of identifying many peptides in a mixture are increased when the complexity of the mixture is decreased. The problem of complexity and how to deal with it can be likened to the problem of printing a book. Imagine printing all the words in this

From: *Introduction to Proteomics: Tools for the New Biology*
By: D. C. Liebler © Humana Press, Inc., Totowa, NJ

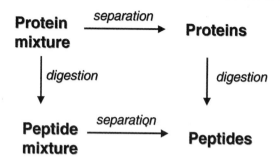

Fig. 1. Protein separation and digestion in proteomics analysis.

book on a single page. It could be done, but the resulting page would be essentially black with ink. By dividing the text onto pages, the complexity is reduced. We can read all the words on one page easily. With protein and peptide separations, we take the same approach. We essentially want to feed the peptide mixture into the MS "a page at a time" to maximize the ability of the instrument to read what is there.

Before we describe different types of protein and peptide separations, it is worth considering how many different proteins and peptides we may be dealing with in a typical proteomic analysis. Based on the number of known human genes, a typical human cell may contain about 20,000 different expressed proteins. If we assume that they average about 50 kDa and contain average numbers of lysine and arginine residues, then each would yield about 30 tryptic peptides. Thus, one cell's proteins would yield about 6,000,000 tryptic peptides. As we will see below, these numbers pose a formidable challenge to even the most efficient multidimensional protein and peptide-separation strategies.

4.3. Extracting Proteins from Biological Samples

In any real study, we start with a biological sample: a piece of tissue, a plate of cultured cells, a flask of bacteria, a leaf, and so on. The sample then is usually pulverized, homogenized, sonicated, or otherwise disrupted to yield a soup that contains cells, subcellular components, and other biological debris in an aqueous buffer or suspension. Proteins are extracted from this soup by a number of techniques. For proteomic analysis, the objective here is to recover as much of the protein as possible with as little contamination by other biomaterials (e.g., lipids, cellulose, nucleic acid, etc.) as possible. This is generally done with the aid of:

- *Detergents* (e.g., SDS, 3-([3-cholamidopropyl]dimethylammonio)-1-propane sulfonate (CHAPS), cholate, Tween), which help to solubilize membrane proteins and aid their separation from lipids
- *Reductants* (e.g., dithiothreitol [DTT], mercaptoethanol, thiourea), which reduce disulfide bonds or prevent protein oxidation
- *Denaturing agents* (e.g., urea and acids), which disrupt protein-protein interactions, secondary and tertiary structures by altering solution ionic strength and pH
- *Enzymes* (e.g., DNAse, RNAse), which digest contaminating nucleic acids, carbohydrates, and lipids.

Investigators in various fields of biology have developed methods to extract proteins from different sample types (e.g, leaves vs cultured cells) and the agents and tricks previously listed are used in different combinations. In some protocols, inhibitors of proteases are commonly used to prevent proteolytic protein degradation. In short, there are many recipes used to extract proteins from biological samples.

One must be aware that some of these agents may interfere with proteomic analysis. For example, phenylmethylsulfonyl fluoride (PMSF), a serine protease inhibitor, is frequently used to prevent protein degradation during tissue processing. However, residual PMSF is some protein samples may inhibit tryptic digestion needed for proteomic analysis. Likewise detergents may interfere both with some analytical protein separations and with proetolytic digestions. Thus, careful attention to the "history" of the sample, particularly how it was harvested and processed, is important to the success of the analytical scheme.

4.4. Protein Separations Before Digestion

In this section, we consider analytical protein separations that are done before the proteins are digested. The three principal separation approaches used with intact proteins are 1D- and 2D-SDS-PAGE and preparative isoelectric focusing (IEF). Although these are most widely used, there are alternatives, particularly HPLC (reverse phase (RP), size exclusion, ion exchange, or affinity chromatography). Regardless of the method used, the idea behind separating intact proteins is to take advantage of their diversity in physical properties, especially isoelectric point and molecular weight. The mixture may be separated into a relatively small number of fractions (as in 1D-SDS-PAGE and preparative IEF) or into many fractions (as in the many spots in 2D-SDS-PAGE). The fractions then are taken for proteolytic digestion followed either by further separation of the peptide fragments or direct MS analysis of the peptides.

4.5. One-Dimensional SDS-PAGE

The single most widely used analytical separation in all of protein chemistry is reasonably useful for proteomic analysis. In 1D-SDS-PAGE, the protein sample is dissolved in a loading buffer that usually contains a thiol reductant (mercaptoethanol or DTT) and SDS (**Fig. 2**). The separation method is based on the binding of SDS to the protein, which imparts negative charge (from the SDS sulfate group) to the protein in roughly constant proportion to molecular weight. When the gel is subjected to high voltage, the protein-SDS complexes migrate through the cross-linked polyacrylamide gel at rates based on their ability to penetrate the pore matrix of the gel. The proteins thus are resolved into bands in order of molecular weight.

One-dimensional-SDS-PAGE is done on gels in which the extent of cross-linking (i.e., polymerization of the acrylamide) varies from 5–15%, where lower degrees of cross-linking allow easier passage of larger proteins through the gel. One can choose an extent of cross-linking based on expected characteristics of the proteins in the sample. For example, a sample containing low molecular-weight proteins is better resolved on a more highly cross-linked gel. Alternatively, one may choose a gradient gel, where the extent of cross-linking increases from top to bottom of the gel. Gradient gels can provide better resolution of a broad molecular-weight range of proteins.

The degree of resolution achieved by 1D-SDS-PAGE is rather modest and bands that appear to contain a single protein may actually contain multiple molecular species. For example, a gel slice spanning an approx 5 kDa range from a crude cellular extract may contain from

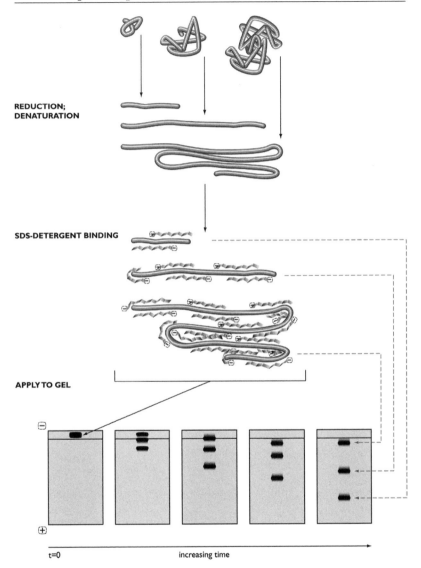

Fig. 2. Schematic representation of 1D-SDS-PAGE.

dozens to hundreds of different proteins. Even a "purified protein" may contain diverse molecular forms. This is often clearly evident when one compares 1D- and 2D-SDS-PAGE of protein samples. The 1D-SDS-PAGE analysis will often give a single, clean-looking band, whereas 2D-SDS-PAGE of the same sample will resolve the sample into multiple spots along the same molecular-weight band, but with different isoelectric points. This can reflect multiple posttranslational modifications that do not significantly affect SDS binding or migration through the polyacrylamide gel.

As the goal of the protein separations is to reduce the complexity of the mixture, it might seem from the aforementioned that 1D-SDS-PAGE is of little utility in proteomic analysis. Actually, the utility of this separation approach depends on the complexity of the sample. Most 1D-SDS-PAGE separations distribute proteins over a lane of between 5 and 15 cm in length, which then permits slicing of the gel into 5–50 bands without difficulty. For a highly complex protein mixture, such as a whole-cell extract, each fraction (gel slice) may still contain many different proteins and the degree of simplification of the sample is only modest. However, many samples for proteomic analysis will not be whole-cell extracts or similarly complex mixtures. For example, proteomics approaches to studying protein-protein interactions (to be discussed in subsequent chapters) may contain relatively few proteins. Likewise, many biological fluids (e.g., cerebrospinal fluid [CSF], lung-lining fluid) contain a much more limited number of proteins and a 1D-SDS-PAGE separation may be quite appropriate to pre-resolving these mixtures.

4.6. Two-Dimensional SDS-PAGE

This separation method has become synonymous with proteomics and remains the single best method for resolving highly complex protein mixtures. Two-dimensional SDS-PAGE is actually a combination of two different types of separations. In the first, the proteins are resolved on the basis of isoelectric point by IEF. In the second, focused proteins then are further resolved by electrophoresis on a polyacrylamide gel (**Fig. 3**). Thus 2D-SDS-PAGE resolves proteins in the first dimension by isoelectric point and in the second dimension by molecular weight.

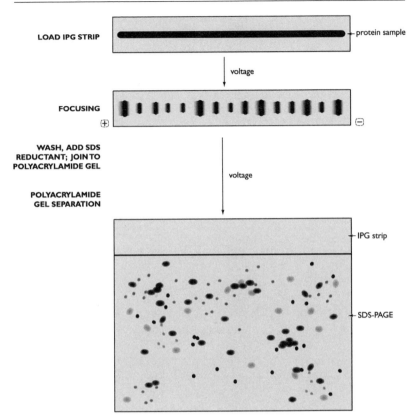

LOAD IPG STRIP   ← protein sample

voltage

FOCUSING

⊕   ⊖

WASH, ADD SDS
REDUCTANT; JOIN TO
POLYACRYLAMIDE GEL

voltage

POLYACRYLAMIDE
GEL SEPARATION

← IPG strip

← SDS-PAGE

Fig. 3. Schematic representation of 2D-SDS-PAGE.

Although 2D-SDS-PAGE is the most effective means of resolving complex protein mixtures, it was not widely used for many years after it was first introduced in the early 1970s. This reflected: 1) the relative technical difficulty of performing the IEF step, and 2) getting the focused proteins into the SDS-PAGE gel. In its original incarnation, the IEF step relied on "tube gels," which were tricky to set up and run. Moreover, the pH gradients in the tube gels were difficult to reproduce. Finally, getting the delicate tube gel containing the focused proteins set up to efficiently transfer the proteins in the SDS-PAGE slab gel was a technical challenge. Thus, 2D-SDS-PAGE was difficult to do and even more difficult to do reproducibly.

This situation has changed much for the better with the introduction of new, dedicated 2D-SDS-PAGE systems that use immobilized pH gradient (IPG) strips and relatively foolproof hardware to facilitate the transfer of proteins from the IPG strip into the SDS-PAGE slab gel. The IPG strip is based on the use of immobilized pH gradients, in which polycarboxylic acid ampholytes are immobilized on supports to reproducibly create stable pH gradients. One can now purchase IPG strips from major suppliers that afford reproducible separations over a variety of wide and narrow pH ranges. The use of narrow pH ranges facilitates the separation of proteins with highly similar isoelectric points. The steps in an IEF separation are summarized in **Fig. 3**. The strip is hydrated with a buffer and the protein is slowly loaded into the strip under voltage. Then the voltage is increased to achieve focusing. Commercially available systems provide temperature control as well as highly accurate voltage or current control to facilitate reproducible separations.

After the focusing step, the strip is treated with a buffer that contains a thiol reductant and SDS and then is joined to the SDS-PAGE slab gel. In this respect, the IPG strip containing the focused proteins acts as a "stacking" gel in 1D-SDS-PAGE. The proteins then are resolved on the SDS-PAGE slab gel in the same manner as for 1D-SDS-PAGE.

Proteins separated by 2D gels are visualized by conventional staining techniques, including silver, Coomassie, and amido black stains. Silver-staining and newer fluorescent dyes are the most sensitive. Although there are many different protocols for all of these staining techniques, not all of them are compatible with subsequent analysis of the proteins. For example, silver-staining with formalin fixation of the proteins tends to fix proteins in the gel, preventing both their digestion and the recovery of any peptides formed. Similar problems result from prolonged exposure of gels to acetic acid. Thus, it is important to use staining protocols that are compatible with subsequent digestion and elution steps.

4.7. Problems with 2D-SDS-PAGE

Despite the superiority of 2D-SDS-PAGE over other methods as a means of resolving complex protein mixtures, the technique presents

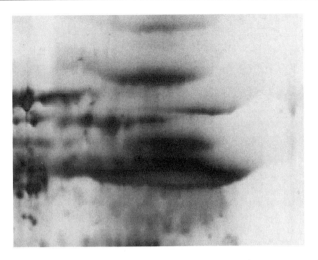

Fig. 4. Section of a 2D gel depicting "smearing" of protein in the IEF (horizontal) direction.

some problems. The first is the difficulty of performing completely reproducible 2D-SDS-PAGE analyses. This problem becomes important when one wishes to use 2D-SDS-PAGE to compare two samples by comparing the images of the stained gels. Differences in protein migration in either dimension could be mistaken for differences in levels of certain proteins between the two samples.

A second problem with 2D-SDS-PAGE is the relative incompatibility of some proteins with the first-dimension IEF step. Many large, hydrophobic proteins simply do not behave well in this type of analysis. Marginal solubility leads to protein precipitation and aggregation, which leads to "smearing" of proteins within the IPG strip, rather than clean focusing into discrete bands. When these proteins are subsequently run in the second (SDS-PAGE) dimension, these proteins appear as streaks across a molecular-weight region (**Fig. 4**). A related issue may be considered either an advantage or a disadvantage of 2D-SDS-PAGE, depending on one's point of view. IEF of proteins often resolves proteins into multiple, discrete bands due to the presence of multiple protein forms with different isoelectric points. For example, deamidation, which converts neutral amides to anionic carboxyl groups can change the protein's pI and its migration in the

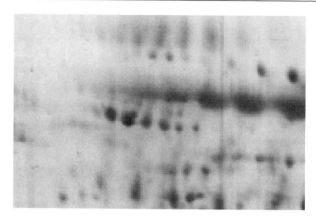

Fig. 5. Section of a 2D gel depicting "spot trains" due to differently modified/charged forms of the same protein.

IPG strip. Other modifications that may affect pI include glycosylation, phosphorylation, oxidation, and exogenous chemical modifications. In some cases, differently modified variants of the same polypeptide may appear as spot "trains" (**Fig. 5**). Although this degree of resolution can be useful in establishing what different protein forms are present, it can also complicate the problem of estimating relative protein expression in two samples by 2D-SDS-PAGE.

A third problem with 2D-SDS-PAGE is the relatively small dynamic range of protein staining as a detection technique. Spot densities reflect about a 100-fold range of protein concentrations, at best. This means that staining of 2D-gels allows the visualization of abundant proteins, whereas less abundant proteins frequently cannot be detected. An excellent example comes from the work of Steven Gygi and Ruedi Aebersold, who studied the relationship of gene expression (measured by mRNA transcripts) and protein levels (measured by incorporation of radiolabeled methionine) in yeast. Yeast express about two-thirds of their ~6000 genes, yet careful 2D-SDS-PAGE analysis with visualization by silver-staining revealed a maximum of about 1000 proteins. In other words, of about 4000 expressed genes, 3000 were *not* detected in the 2D-SDS-PAGE analysis. Most of the proteins detected were products of genes with high codon bias values (*see* Chapter 2) and thus with a tendency toward higher expression. Two-dimensional

SDS-PAGE thus tends to be best for analysis of abundant, long-lived proteins. Unfortunately, many proteins of considerable interest in biology are expressed at relatively low levels and are rapidly turned over. For proteomic analysis of these proteins, other analytical approaches are often necessary.

4.8. Preparative IEF

This technique is analogous to the first step in 2D-SDS-PAGE. In preparative IEF, the separation is carried out on an IPG strip, in a tube gel, or in solution. Of these, the latter is most widely used. The generation of a pH gradient is achieved with soluble ampholytes, which are polycarboxylic acid compounds that generate a stable pH gradient when voltage is applied across the focusing cell. The protein sample then is added, voltage again is applied, and the proteins then are separated by isoelectric point. In commercially available apparatus, such as the BioRad Rotofor™ cell, the focusing cell is divided by permeable membranes into a series of chambers. After the focusing step, the chambers are quickly and simultaneously emptied by a vacuum sipper that draws the contents of each section of the cell into a separate tube. With this type of apparatus, the entire protein mixture is separated into 12–20 fractions.

An advantage of the solution phase isoelectric focusing is the relatively large sample capacity (milligrams to grams of total protein per run) and the relative ease of working with samples in solutions as opposed to gels. The ampholytes can be removed from the fractionated samples by dialysis or gel filtration prior to further processing of the proteins. Recovery of proteins from solution-phase IEF typically exceeds 85–90%. Detergents and chaotropic agents can be used to maintain solubility of hydrophobic proteins. As with the IEF step in 2D-SDS-PAGE, this separation takes advantage of the diversity in physical properties (in this case, pI) of intact proteins. However, working with diverse intact proteins also carries disadvantages, such as the tendency of some proteins to aggregate and precipitate during solution-phase focusing.

4.9. High-Performance Liquid Chromatography

Availability of improved stationary-phase materials and hardware has greatly improved the performance of LC systems for protein purification. Although HPLC of intact proteins has not become a widely used technique for analytical proteomics, it is nevertheless highly applicable as an initial step to fractionate protein mixtures. Diverse chromatographic separations are available, including RP, anion and cation exchange, size exclusion, and affinity chromatography. The latter is particularly attractive as a means of pulling a subset of proteins from a complex mixture.

HPLC would appear to be about as useful as preparative IEF for resolving protein mixtures into fractions. The advantage of HPLC is the diversity of separation modes available. Indeed, tandem HPLC separations combine two different types of chromatography. For example, strong cation exchange, followed by RP, would apply two completely different separation modes. As we will discuss regarding the HPLC of peptides, ion exchange can be coupled in series to RP chromatography to achieve highly effective tandem LC separations.

4.10. Protein Separations After Digestion

In this approach, the proteins in the sample are first digested into a mixture of peptides, then the peptides are separated prior to analysis. The extreme application of this approach would be to digest a complete cell or tissue extract to peptides and then perform MS analysis on the mixture. Indeed, this sort of analysis has been done with considerable success. The use of microcapillary HPLC with special control adaptations and automated MS instrument control (all discussed later in this book) allowed the acquisition of MS data on hundreds or thousands of peptides in a single run. The primary rationale for this approach is that it permits one to convert a very heterogeneous mixture of proteins to a more homogeneous mixture of peptides, which can be more easily analyzed. If one does elect this approach, the number of available methods to separate peptide mixtures is far more limited. One-dimensional- and 2D-SDS-PAGE are out, as they are not practically useful in resolving peptides from digests, which typically display a much more limited range of pI and molecular weight. Although it can be performed on peptide mixtures, preparative IEF may be of limited utility for resolving peptide mixtures. However, little has been done to evaluate preparative IEF as a tool for peptide separations and it cannot be ruled out.

4.11. Tandem LC Approaches for Peptide Analysis

Certainly the most widely used approach to analysis of peptide mixtures is HPLC. As noted earlier in the discussion of separations of intact proteins, the diversity of stationary phases and separation modes gives HPLC considerable resolving power. The combination of HPLC separation modes is one of the most effective tools in analytical proteomics. The use of combined separation modes in series is referred to as "tandem HPLC." The idea behind tandem LC is that the combination of dissimilar separation modes allows a greater resolution of peptides in a mixture. Consider the major HPLC separation modes and the characteristics that dictate separation.

- RP: hydrophobicity
- Strong cation exchange: net positive charge
- Strong anion exchange: net negative charge
- Size exclusion: peptide size/molecular weight
- Affinity: interaction with specific functional groups

Of the separation modes listed here, all but size exclusion are likely to be useful for peptide separations. The resolving power of available size-exclusion media is not sufficient to separate peptides in the molecular-weight range that results from proteolytic digests.

John Yates and colleagues have effectively exploited tandem LC-MS to analyze complex peptide mixtures. Their approach employed microcapillary columns linked in series and eluted directly into the mass spectrometer (**Fig. 6**). They coined the term "MudPIT" (Multidimensional Protein Identification Technique) to describe the approach. Peptides are first applied to a strong cation exchange (SCX) column, which serves as the "front end" of the system (**Fig. 7**). Peptides adsorb to the SCX column with affinities that are proportional to the overall number of positive charges (e.g., ionized nitrogens) on each peptide. The peptides are eluted by a step gradient of increasing salt concentration. Each step releases a group of peptides, which then pass on the RP column, which is downstream of the SCX column. Each peptide group then is separated by a RP-HPLC gradient, which resolves the peptides on the basis of their hydrophobicity. From the RP column, the peptides pass directly into the MS instrument for

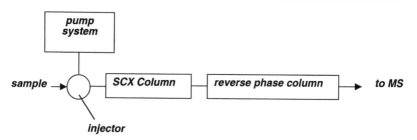

Fig. 6. Schematic of tandem ion exchange (SCX)-RP-HPLC system.

analysis. After the RP gradient is complete, the next step of the salt gradient releases more peptides from the SCX column, which then are further resolved by the RP column prior to passage into the MS. This cycle is continued until all of the peptides have been eluted from the SCX column.

In comparing the MudPIT tandem LC approach to RP-HPLC alone for LC-MS, it is clear that the tandem approach greatly increased the number of peptides that were identified in a single run. As discussed earlier, the tandem approach serves to further "spread out" the peptide mixture, so that the MS can obtain data on a greater fraction of the components. In addition, the tandem LC approach also facilitated the identification of peptides from proteins that were present in the mixture at low abundance. Analyses of yeast proteins by the MudPIT approach revealed a significantly improved identification of peptides from low-abundance proteins. This is in contrast to 2S-SDS-PAGE, which tended to identify more highly expressed proteins.

The superiority of tandem LC over 2D-SDS-PAGE probably is owing to two factors, one obvious and the other not so obvious. First, proteins are selected from 2D gels for digestion and MS only if they can be visualized by staining. However, the limits of detection of many MS instruments are below the levels at which proteins can be detected by gel staining. Thus, if one cannot see a protein spot to harvest and analyze, no data will be collected on that protein. Second, handling of proteins in mixtures may provide a "carrier effect," in which the presence of more abundant peptides prevents the loss of less abundant peptides. When one works with very dilute samples with little material (such as would be obtained from a very weak 2D gel

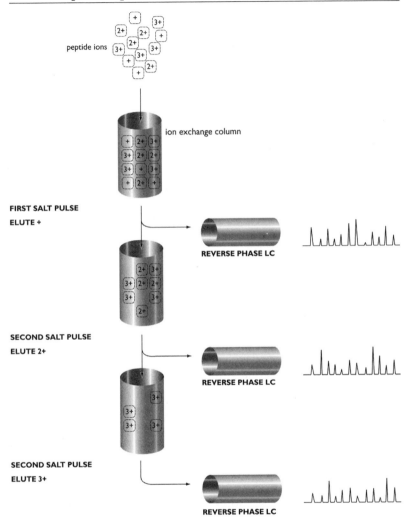

Fig. 7. Multistage fractionation of a peptide mixture by in-line strong cation exchange and RP-HPLC.

spot), the fractional loss due to interaction with surfaces and other processing components is relatively high. In the presence of larger amounts of other peptides in a more complex mixture, the other, more abundant peptides also adsorb to the surfaces in the system and reduce the loss of the less abundant components.

It would appear that other combinations of LC separation modes would also be useful. Possibilities include strong anion exchange/RP and affinity/RP-HPLC. The application of tandem LC to proteomic analysis is relatively new and this promising approach will certainly undergo increasing development and become much more widely used.

4.12. Capillary Electrophoresis

Capillary electrophoresis (CE) operates on the same general principal as IEF. Proteins placed in an electric field will migrate to a point in a pH gradient where they display an overall neutral change. The performance of the analysis in a microcapillary tube provides greatly enhanced resolution over the preparative IEF techniques discussed earlier. CE offers the greatest resolution of all peptide analytical techniques and can be coupled directly to MS instruments. CE thus has great potential as a technique for analytical proteomics. The utility of CE is limited at the present time by the lack of commercially available, robust, and reliable CE-MS instrumentation for analytical proteomics. Development of instrumentation for this purpose is continuing and CE-MS may become a very useful tool in proteomics analysis in the near future.

4.13. Which Approach is Best?

The use of an initial protein separation followed by digestion and analysis is the most widely practiced analytical proteomics approach today. This is based largely on the preeminence of 2S-SDS-PAGE for protein separations. The biggest single advantage of this approach is the ability of 2D gels to serve as image maps to allow investigators to compare changes in the proteome based on changes in the patterns of spots on the gel. As noted earlier, there are several factors that can confound interpretations of 2D gel-spot patterns. Nevertheless, there is no other technique available that provides an intuitive "snapshot" of the proteome. For this reason, 2D-SDS-PAGE is likely to remain

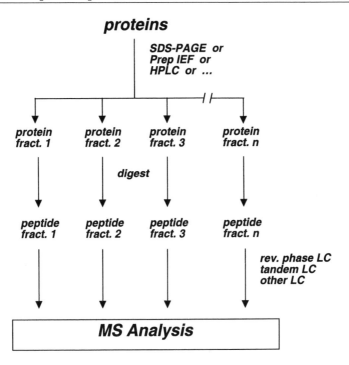

Fig. 8. Generic approach to protein/peptide fractionation.

a dominant methodology in proteomics. Nevertheless, for lower-abundance proteins, 2D gels will not prove useful, simply because important proteins cannot be seen. In this case, other separation methods, particularly tandem LC, provide a viable alternative.

Based on all the considerations discussed earlier, the most flexible, comprehensive strategy for proteome characterization may be a hybrid of methods. A generic hybrid approach is depicted in **Fig. 8**. In the first step, proteins first are separated as intact species, either by preparative IEF, preparative 1D-SDS-PAGE, or HPLC. The fractions obtained from these separations then are subjected to enzymatic digestion and the resulting peptides are subject to HPLC separations prior to introduction into the MS. Depending on the complexity of the original sample or the goals of the analysis, the HPLC separation may involve a single separation mode (e.g., RP) or a tandem LC separation. A key advantage of this generic approach is its overall flexibility and ease of adaptation to instrumentation available in different laboratories. Another advantage of the approach is that the front-end protein separations are capable of handling relatively large amounts of protein (many mg in most cases). Thus, the possibility of detecting low-abundance components as peptides in the final MS analysis is improved. Although the feasibility of several variants of this generic approach has been documented by recent work, further work will be needed to more clearly establish which variations are the least troublesome, most efficient, and most reliable.

Suggested Reading

Gygi, S. P., Corthnls, G. L., Zhang, Y., Rochon, Y. and Aebersold, R. (2000) Evaluation of two-dimensional gel electrophoresis-based proteome analysis technology. *Proc. Nat. Acad. Sci.* **97,** 9390–9395.

Link, A. J. (1998) *2-D Proteome Analysis Protocols.* Humana Press, Totowa, NJ.

Link, A. J., Eng, J., Schieltz, D. M., Carmack, E., Mize, G. J., Morris, D. R., et al. (1999) Direct analysis of protein complexes using mass spectrometry. *Nat. Biotechnol.* **17,** 676–682.

Rabilloud, T. (2000) Detecting proteins separated by 2D gel electrophoresis. *Anal. Chem.* **72,** 48A–55A.

Walker, J. M. (1996) *Protein Protocols Handbook.* Humana Press, Totowa, NJ.

Wall, D. B., Kachman, M. T., Gong, S., Hinderer, R., Parus, S., Misek, D. E., et al. (2000) Isoelectric focusing nonporous RP HPLC: a two-dimensional liquid-phase separation method for mapping of cellular proteins with identification using MALDI-TOF mass spectrometry. *Anal. Chem.* **72,** 1099–1111.

Washburn, M. P., Wolters, D., and Yates, J. R. (2001) Large-scale analysis of the yeast proteome by multidimensional protein identification technology. *Nat. Biotechnol.* **19,** 242–247.

5 Protein Digestion Techniques

5.1. Why Digest Proteins?

Modern MS instruments are capable of measuring the molecular weights of intact proteins with a fairly high degree of accuracy. So why not do proteomics simply by measuring the masses of intact proteins? Unfortunately, intact mass measurements are of relatively little use for three reasons. First, as good as MS instruments are, there are still errors in the measurements they produce. The greater the mass of the protein, the greater the absolute magnitude of the error. Those errors introduce enough uncertainty to make the measurements insufficiently accurate for definitive identification. Moreover, diverse posttranslational modifications further complicate assignments based on mass. Second, not all proteins are amenable to intact mass measurements. It can be very difficult to obtain mass measurements on very large and hydrophobic proteins. Third, the sensitivity of measurements of intact protein masses is not nearly as good as sensitivity for peptide mass measurements and peptide tandem MS analyses. For these reasons, doing proteomics by analyzing intact proteins is not a realistic option at present.

There are two other reasons why analysis of peptides, rather than proteins, is the approach of choice. MS instruments now are well-suited to the analysis of peptides. As we shall see in the next chapter, modern MS instruments can perform highly accurate mass measurements

From: *Introduction to Proteomics: Tools for the New Biology*
By: D. C. Liebler © Humana Press, Inc., Totowa, NJ

of peptides and can also obtain data from which peptide sequence can be deduced with certainty. Moreover, the data obtained from MS analysis of peptides can be taken directly for comparison to protein sequences derived from protein and nucleotide-sequence databases. A key element of the search algorithms that assign protein identity from comparisons of peptide MS data to database information is the knowledge that certain proteolytic enzymes cleave the proteins to peptides at specific sites. In the remainder of this chapter, we will look at the enzymes and approaches to generate peptides from proteins for MS analysis.

5.2. What Do We Want Digestion to Accomplish?

The ideal protein digestion approach would cleave proteins at certain specific amino acid residues to yield fragments that are most compatible with MS analysis. Specifically, peptide fragments of between about 6–20 amino acids are ideal for MS analysis and database comparisons. Peptides shorter than about 6 amino acids generally are too short to produce unique sequence matches in database searches. On the other hand, it is difficult to obtain sequence information from peptides longer than 20 amino acids in tandem MS analyses (this point will be discussed in more detail in the next chapter). Thus, the objective of protein digestion will be to produce the highest yield of peptides of optimal length for MS analysis.

5.3. Overview of Proteases

Nature has evolved a diverse collection of proteases to undertake the endless tasks of protein remodeling that are essential to higher organisms. Although thousands of distinct proteases have been purified or characterized, most are available only in limited quantities, and only to those protease biochemists who can purify or express them. What is really needed for analytical proteomics are stable, well-characterized enzymes with well-defined specificities. These enzymes must be available in quantity and high purity and must be robust enough for application in a variety of circumstances. A number of proteases that meet these requirements have been

Table 1
Proteases and Their Cleavage Specificities

Enzyme	Cleavage specificity
Trypsin	/K-, /R-, \P
Chymotrypsin	/W-, /Y-, /F-, \P
Glu C (V8 protease)	/E-, /D^a-, \P
Lys C	/K-, \P
Asp N	/D-

^{a}Cleavage after aspartate and glutamate in sodium phosphate buffer; otherwise cleavage only after glutamate.

used for proteomic analysis. **Table 1** summarizes the proteases that are most widely used in proteomic analyses and their cleavage characteristics. The following sections provide short summaries of the major characteristics of the enzymes.

5.4. Trypsin

Trypsin is by far the most widely used protease in proteomic analysis. This well-characterized serine protease displays several of the desired characteristics enumerated above. Trypsin is obtained primarily from porcine or bovine pancreas and is easily purified. It can be obtained modified with tosylphenylalanylchloromethane (TCPK) to inhibit residual chymotrypsin. Trypsin cleaves proteins at lysine and arginine residues, unless either of these is followed by a proline residue in the C-terminal direction. The spacing of lysine and arginine residues in many proteins is such that many of the resulting peptides are of a length well-suited to MS analysis. This "dual specificity" means that trypsin will cut proteins more frequently than will a protease that cuts at only one amino acid residue. As a general rule, a 50 kDa protein will yield about 30 tryptic peptides.

An advantage of trypsin for proteomics work is that the enzyme displays good activity both in solution and in "in gel" digestion protocols (*see* below). A number of protocols for trypsin digestions or proteins in solution, in gels, and on membrane blots have been developed and have been widely tested. Moreover, MS laboratories that routinely carry out proteomics analyses frequently are familiar with trypsin autolysis fragments, which inevitably appear as by-products of tryptic-digestion protocols.

5.5. Glu-C (V8-protease)

Glu-C is an endoproteinase that cleaves at the carboxyl side of glutamate residues in either ammonium acetate or ammonium bicarbonate buffer. In a sodium phosphate buffer, however, the enzyme cleaves at both glutamate and aspartate residues. Glu-C can be used for in-gel digestions. An advantage of using Glu-C is that it displays a markedly different cleavage specificity than trypsin, which improves the likelihood to obtaining complementary peptide fragments of a protein. This can be particularly useful, for example, for analysis of proteins with regions of high lysine and arginine content. These regions may undergo extensive cleavage with trypsin to yield very short peptides with little or no sequence context.

5.6. Other Proteases and Cleavage Reagents

Several other enzymes are used for proteomic analysis. These include Lys-C, chymotrypsin, Asp-N, and several "nonspecific" proteases. The cleavage specificity of these enzymes generally is not ideal for most proteomic analyses. Those enzymes that cleave at only one amino acid residue tend to yield fewer, larger fragments that do not provide useful sequence information is tandem MS analyses. On the other hand, chymotrypsin may cleave too frequently (based on its ability to cleave at tyrosine, phenylalanine, and tryptophan) to yield too many small pepides that lack adequate sequence context. Nevertheless, these proteases are often useful in specific situations, where the sequence of a protein of interest does not yield satisfactory tryptic peptides, particularly in some region of interest.

5.7. Nonspecific Proteases

Another potentially useful strategy in protein digestion is the use of nonspecific proteases, such as subtilysin, pepsin, proteinase K, and pronase. These enzymes cleave proteins more or less randomly to produce multiple overlapping peptides. Because of the relative lack of specificity, digestions must be carried out for relatively short periods of time to prevent them from going too far. However, the advantage

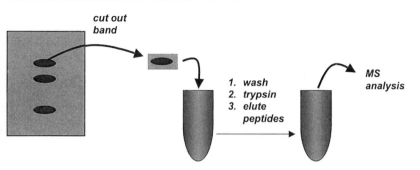

Fig. 1. Schematic representation of in-gel digestion.

of producing multiple overlapping peptides is that they increase the liklihood of obtaining sequence data over a greater percentage of each protein analyzed.

5.8. Cyanogen Bromide

Proteins also can be cleaved with some chemicals. The most widely used of these is cyanogen bromide (CNBr), which cleaves proteins at methionine residues. Although the reaction proceeds with a high degree of specificity, the relative infrequency of methionine residues in most proteins means that CNBr cleavage yields relatively few, large fragments. In many cases, these large fragments do not yield useful sequence data in tandem MS analyses.

5.9. In-Gel Digestions

A commonly used approach to digestion of proteins separated by 1D- or 2D-SDS-PAGE is referred to as "in-gel" digestion (**Figure 1**). The band or spot of interest is cut from the gel, destained, and then treated with a protease (most commonly trypsin). The enzyme penetrates the gel matrix and digests the protein to peptides, which then are eluted from the gel by washing. This technique is an indispensable element to 2D-SDS-PAGE proteomics strategies.

Although trypsin is the most commonly used enzyme, the general approach is applicable to other proteases, including Glu C and chymotrypsin. The efficiency of both digestion and recovery of peptides from the gels is highly variable. A key determinant of successful in-gel digestions is the gel-staining technique used. Staining protocols that employ aldehyde fixatives or prolonged exposure to acids (e.g., acetic acid) tend to fix proteins in gels, thus making the proteins difficult to digest and the peptides difficult to elute. With highly cross-linked gels, the penetration of protease enzymes into the gel matrix may be retarded. Finally, residual components of the SDS-PAGE technique (SDS or residual unpolymerized acrylamide) may be inhibitory to protease activities.

Analogous protocols can be used for "on blot" digestion of proteins that have been blotted onto nitrocellulose or polyvinylidenefluoride (PVDF) membranes. As with in-gel digestions, the section of membrane containing the proteins of interest are cut out and subjected to digestion with a protease, followed by elution from the membrane surface.

Suggested Reading

Jensen, O. N., Wilm, M., Shevchenko, A., and Mann, M. (1999) Sample preparation methods for mass spectrometric peptide mapping directly from 2-DE gels. *Methods Mol. Biol.* **112,** 513–530.

Shevchenko, A., Wilm, M., Vorm, O., and Mann, M. (1996) Mass spectrometric sequencing of proteins silver-stained polyacrylamide gels. *Anal. Chem.* **68,** 850–858.

Walker, J. M. (1996) *Protein Protocols Handbook.* Humana Press, Totowa, NJ.

6 Mass Spectrometers for Protein and Peptide Analysis

6.1. Introduction

Two different types of instruments are used for most proteomics MS work: the MALDI-TOF instruments and the ESI-tandem MS instruments. The two types operate in entirely different ways and generate different, but complementary information. Indeed, the best-equipped proteomics laboratories have both types of instruments available. This chapter describes how each of these instruments works and what types of data they produce, and compares them on the basis of their advantages and limitations. Before we get to the instruments themselves, let's take a look at the basics of MS instrumentation.

6.2. How MS Instruments Work

Mass spectrometers have three essential parts (**Fig. 1**). The first is the *source*, which produces ions from the sample. The second is the *mass analyzer*, which resolves ions based on their mass/charge (m/z) ratio. The third part is the *detector*, which detects the ions resolved by the mass analyzer. In short, the mass spectrometer converts components of a mixture to ions and then analyzes them on the basis of their m/z. The data are automatically recorded by the data system and can then be retrieved for manual or computer-assisted interpretation.

Of course, there is more to the functioning MS system. Modern MS instruments are controlled by sophisticated computers and software and the data the instruments generate are handled by similarly

From: *Introduction to Proteomics: Tools for the New Biology*
By: D. C. Liebler © Humana Press, Inc., Totowa, NJ

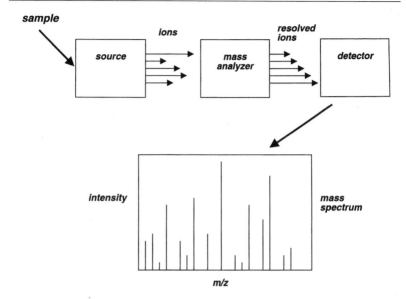

Fig. 1. Schematic representation of a mass spectrometer.

sophisticated computer data systems. The instruments also are equipped with vacuum-pump systems to maintain the mass analyzers and detectors at high vacuum, which is required for their function. In contrast to MS instruments of yesteryear, today's MS instruments are relatively small, compact, reliable, and, best of all, easy to use.

6.3. What Do We Want from MS Data?

For purposes of proteomics, we want good data on peptide masses (MALDI-TOF MS) or good data that describe peptide fragmentation (ESI tandem MS). So what makes good data? We look for three things. The first is sensitivity. As noted earlier, in much proteomics work, the amounts of proteins are limited. Thus, we need instruments that are routinely capable of obtaining data on femtomole (10^{-15} mole) quantities of peptides or less. Second, we need *resolution*, which is the measure of how well we can distinguish ions of very similar m/z values. The MS instruments that deliver the highest resolution (magnetic sector instruments or fourier transform instruments) can reliably distinguish between ions that differ in m/z by as little as 0.001 amu. However, these expensive, temperamental instruments are not routinely used in proteomics work. Instruments commonly used in MS need to be able to distinguish ions differing in m/z values of at least one Da (i.e., the mass of a single hydrogen atom). The ability of some mass analyzers to provide greater resolution can be useful in specific situations, as will be discussed later. Finally, we need *mass accuracy*. This means that the measured values for peptide ions or their fragment ions must as close as possible to their real values. This is particularly important when we use the data to identify peptides based on comparisons with (real) database values.

6.4. MALDI-TOF MS Instruments

MALDI-TOF is the standard acronym for matrix-assisted laser desorption ionization-time of flight. The first part (MALDI) refers to the source, whereas the TOF refers to the mass analyzer. The term "MALDI" actually describes a method of ionization, but frequently is used in the proteomics literature as shorthand for MALDI-TOF. However, both MALDI sources and TOF analyzers can be used in other configurations.

6.5. How the MALDI Source Works

To understand how a MALDI-TOF instrument works, it is easiest to start with the MALDI source (**Fig. 2A**). The sample to be analyzed is mixed with a chemical *matrix*, which typically contains a small organic molecule with a desirable chromophore that absorbs light at a specific wavelength. Typical matrix compounds include 2,5-dihydroxybenzoic acid, 3,5-dimethoxy-4-hydroxycinnamic acid (sinapinic acid), and α-cyano-4-hydroxycinnamic acid. The admixture of sample and matrix is then spotted onto a small plate or slide and then allowed to evaporate in air. The evaporation of residual water or other solvent from the sample allows the formation of a crystal lattice into which the peptide sample is integrated. The target is then placed into the source. The source is equipped with a laser, which fires a beam of light at the target. The matrix chemicals absorb photons from the beam and become electronically excited. This excess energy is then transferred to the peptides or proteins in the sample, which are then ejected from the target surface into the gas phase.

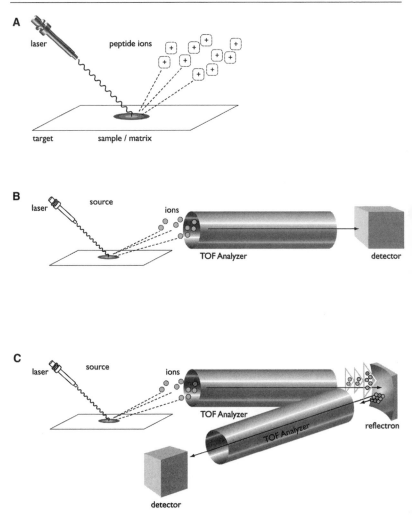

Fig. 2. Schematic representation of a MALDI-TOF mass spectrometer. **(A)** The MALDI ionization process. **(B)** A MALDI-TOF instrument operating in linear mode. **(C)** A MALDI-TOF instrument equipped with a reflectron.

This ionization process produces both positive and negative ions, depending on the nature of the sample. For peptides and proteins, the positive ions are almost always the species of interest. The positive ions are formed by accepting a proton as they are ejected from the matrix. Each peptide molecule tends to pick up a single proton. Thus, most of the resulting peptide ions are *singly charged*. For a peptide of mass 1032, the addition of a proton and its one positive charge makes the m/z value 1033 for the $[M+H]^+$ ion. The ions formed in the MALDI source are then extracted and directed into the TOF mass analyzer.

6.6. The TOF Mass Analyzer

The TOF (time of flight) mass analyzer works just like its name sounds. The TOF analyzer measures the time it takes for the ions to fly from one end of the analyzer to the other and strike the detector. The speed with which the ions fly down the analyzer tube is proportional to their m/z values. The greater the m/z, the faster they fly.

The first TOF analyzers worked in just this simple way (**Fig. 2B**). These simple start-to-finish analyzers operated in what is referred to as "linear mode." The ions were formed in the MALDI source, continually extracted from the source, and then sent down the flight tube to the detector. Unfortunately, the resolution of instruments running in linear mode with continuous extraction of ions was relatively poor. Resolution in mass spectrometry refers to the ability of the instrument to distinguish between ions of slightly different m/z values. MS resolution can be likened to visual focus; poor resolution is like nearsightedness. The lack of resolution in linear-mode instruments is due to variations in the velocities of ions of the same m/z as they fly down the flight tube.

This problem was solved with two important technical innovations. The first is the reflectron, which, according to the visual analogy, acts as a pair of contact lenses for the nearsighted TOF. The reflectron focuses ions of the same m/z values and allows them to reach the detector at the same time (**Fig. 2C**). The reflectron dramatically improved resolution of TOF analyzers. The effect of the reflectron on resolution is vividly illustrated by the spectra in **Fig. 3**. In **Fig. 3B**, a spectrum of insulin obtained in linear mode indicates the average m/z value of the peptide analyzed. In **Fig. 3A**, analysis on an instrument

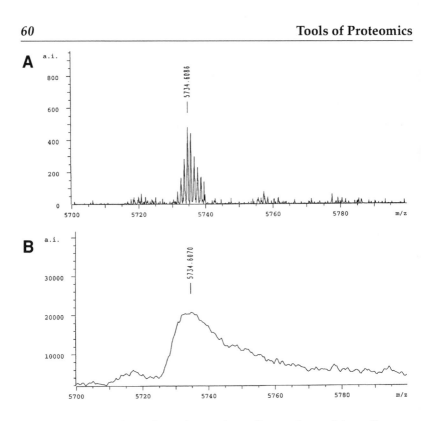

Fig. 3. MALDI-TOF MS analysis of insulin performed in reflectron mode **(A)** and linear mode **(B)**.

with a reflectron easily resolves the individual ions due to the all ^{12}C and the various ^{13}C isotopomers of the peptide.

Another approach to improving the resolution of TOF analyzers in linear mode is the use of pulsed-laser ionization with delayed extraction. The delayed extraction technique involves building a slight delay between the laser pulse (ionization) and the direction of the ions down the flight tube. This permits the ions all to get a "fair start," such that all species of the same m/z will hit the detector at the same time. Spectra are obtained by averaging the spectra obtained from many laser pulses (typically 10–100). The effect of delayed extraction on spectral resolution is similar to that of a reflectron.

The development of TOF analyzer technology has produced some of the best mass analyzers available today. The resolution of the best TOF analyzers is such that peptide ions with m/z differences of 0.001 amu can be reliably distinguished. As we shall see in the next chapter, high resolution and mass accuracy are essential to the reliable application of MALDI-TOF data to protein identification.

Although MALDI-TOF instruments are used in proteomics primarily to obtain mass measurements of intact peptide ions, some instruments can analyze fragmentation of peptide ions as well. A technique called "post-source decay" (PSD) can be used on instruments equipped with a reflectron. In this technique, the voltage on the reflectron is modulated during analysis to allow the detection of fragments of peptide ions formed during ionization and acceleration down the flight tube. Although it is probably not the best MS technique for peptide-sequence analysis, it can frequently be a useful adjunct to measurement of intact peptide masses. One useful aspect of PSD spectra of peptides is the appearance of peptide immonium ions of the general formula $H_2N^+ = CHR$, where R is the amino acid side chain. These immonium ions are indicators of the presence of specific amino acids and can be used with some software tools to help identify peptide sequences.

6.7. Pros and Cons of MALDI

There is no perfect MS instrument for analytical proteomics, but MALDI-TOF MS deserves very high marks in four important categories. First, it is very easy. The instruments are, for the most part, very user-friendly and robust. MALDI-TOF instruments are among the easiest of MS instruments to operate, in large part because there is no HPLC-MS interface to worry about. These instruments are generally very compatible with "walk-up" or "open access" formats in which the system is available on a walk-in basis for routine use by a number of users. Thus, a MALDI-TOF instrument in a shared proteomics facility can easily be set up to handle hundreds of analyses per day.

Second, the MALDI-TOF instruments most widely used today are compatible with new robotic sample preparation devices designed to aid high-throughput proteomics work. With some integrated systems now available, 2D gels are prepared and imaged, the protein spots harvested and digested, and the digests are applied to multisample MALDI targets for analysis, all by robotic devices. This integration not only reduces the labor involved in high-throughput proteomic analysis, but also increases the speed and reproducibility of analyses.

Third, as the accuracy and resolution of TOF analyzers has improved, so has their usefulness in generating useful proteomics data. As we'll see in the next chapter, a critical requirement of reliable protein identification by peptide mass mapping with MALDI-TOF data is good mass measurements for peptides. Today's generation of MALDI-TOF instruments is well-suited to this demanding task.

Finally, MALDI-TOF MS is very sensitive. MALDI-TOF instruments routinely can deliver quality MS data on low femtomole quantities of peptides and the best instruments are capable of attomole (10^{-18} mole) or better sensitivity under optimum conditions. New developments in instrumentation should bring further improvements in sensitivity, resolution, and mass accuracy.

Given all the praise heaped on MALDI-TOF instruments, there would seem to be little reason to consider using anything else. However, MALDI-TOF does present some drawbacks. First, these instruments are best-suited to measuring peptide masses. This type of information, although useful for protein identification, is nevertheless limited. Peptide ion fragmentation provides true sequence data, which has greater intrinsic value. Unfortunately, MALDI-TOF instruments are not well-suited for producing this type of information. As noted earlier, PSD analysis available on some high-end MALDI-TOF instruments does offer peptide sequence capacity, but it is not a true tandem MS technique (*see* below) and is not as reliable a method of obtaining peptide sequence information as ESI tandem MS.

Second, the success of MALDI-TOF analyses is highly dependent on the quality of the sample. Contamination of the peptide digest sample with significant levels of detergents, buffer salts, metals, or organic modifiers (e.g., DTT, urea, glycerol) may greatly inhibit peptide ionization in the MALDI source. Although these variables can affect virtually any MS analysis, MALDI is particularly sensitive because there is no in-line HPLC system to separate contaminants from the sample. However, MALDI-TOF users have employed successful microscale solid-phase cleanup tools (e.g., ZipTips™) to remove salts and other contaminants.

6.8. ESI Tandem MS Instruments

ESI tandem MS (or ESI-MS-MS) is the standard acronym for electrospray ionization tandem mass spectrometry. ESI refers to the process by which ions are produced in the source of the instrument. Tandem mass spectrometry refers to mass analyzers that are able to perform two-stage (or multistage) mass analyses of ions. Several different types of mass analyzers are used in ESI-MS-MS instruments, most commonly quadrupole, ion trap, and TOF mass analyzers. In some cases, these analyzers are used in various combinations. The versatility of different tandem mass analyzers with ESI sources offers excellent instrumental flexibility in approaching analytical proteomics problems.

6.9. Peptide Ions in Solution

To understand how ESI works, let's start with a quick look at the solution acid-base chemistry of peptides. In contrast to MALDI, in which the sample is a dried, crystalline admixture of peptide sample and matrix, the peptides or proteins to be analyzed by ESI are in aqueous solution. Peptides exist as ions in solution because they contain functional groups whose ionization is controlled by the pH of the solution. Thus, carboxylic acids are protonated (unionized) below pH 3.0 and ionized at pH values above about 5.0. In contrast, N-terminal amines and histidine nitrogens are weak bases that are ionized below pH 7.0. The nitrogen functional groups of lysine and arginine are usually ionized below pH 8.5. This all means that at acidic pH values (i.e., pH 3.5 and below), protonation of the amines will confer overall net positive charge to peptides and proteins. At basic pH, deprotonation of the amines and carboxyl groups confers a more negative overall charge. Fragmentation of peptide ions is favored by positive charges on the peptide ions. Moreover the HPLC chromatographic characteristics of peptides are improved at acidic pH values. For these reasons, ESI of peptides is most commonly done in the positive ion mode to analyze acidic samples.

6.10. Peptide Ion Charge States in ESI

A unique characteristic of ESI is the production of multiply charged ions from proteins and peptides. Many peptides bear multiple proton-accepting sites and can exist as singly charged or multiply charged ions in solution. This is particularly true of peptides derived by tryptic digestion, as they bear lysine or arginine residues at their C-termini as well as N-terminal amino groups, both of which may be protonated in acidic solutions. Indeed, "multiple charging" of proteins and peptides serves the added purpose of forming ions that are within the mass range of the quadrupole and ion-trap mass analyzers, which have more limited mass range than the TOF analyzers. For example, the absolute mass of a singly protonated 20 kDa protein (m/z = 20,001) is well outside the mass range of a quadrupole mass analyzer, which typically extends to 2 kDa or sometimes 4 kDa. However, the typical 20 kDa protein will accept anywhere from 10–30 protons in solution. Thus, for a population of these protein molecules in solution, some will have 20 protons and a m/z of 20,020/20 = 1001, some will have 21 protons and a m/z of 20,021/21 = 953, some will have 19 protons and a m/z of 20,019/19 = 1053, and so on. The ESI mass spectrum of the intact protein appears as a so-called "multicharge envelope," in which all of the different charge states of the protein in solution are represented (**Fig. 4A**). Charge-deconvolution algorithms and software can convert this spectrum to one that represents the actual protein mass (**Fig. 4B**). The existence of many charge states occurs with proteins because these very large molecules have many possible proton acceptors each in equilibrium with the solution.

In contrast to intact proteins, peptides of 250–2500 Da typically exist as a mixture of singly, doubly, and triply charged ions, depending on their sizes and numbers of basic amino acid residues present. For the typical peptide in this mass range, the doubly charged ion is predominant, but singly and triply charged ions frequently can be observed. The distribution of these ions can be seen in the spectrum of the model peptide AVAGCAGAR in **Fig. 5**.

6.11. How the ESI Source Works

The mechanics of the ESI source are relatively simple (**Fig. 6**). The sample enters the source through a flow stream (often from the HPLC) and passes through a stainless-steel cone or needle held at high voltage. As the flow stream exits the needle, it sprays out in a fine mist of droplets. The droplets contain peptide ions as well as components of the HPLC mobile phase (water, acetonitrile, acetic acid,

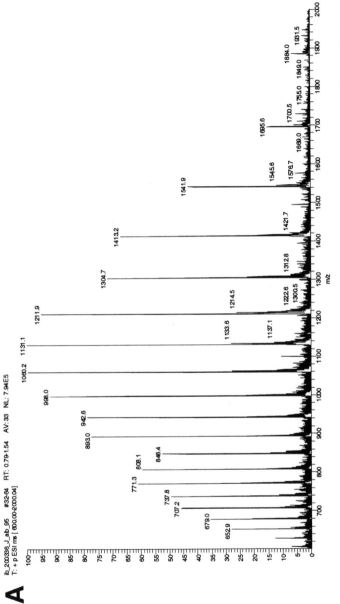
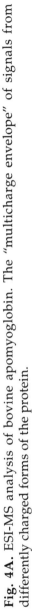

Fig. 4A. ESI-MS analysis of bovine apomyoglobin. The "multicharge envelope" of signals from differently charged forms of the protein.

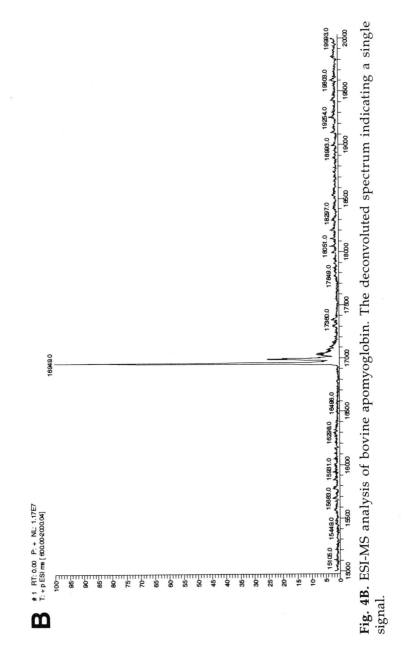

Fig. 4B. ESI-MS analysis of bovine apomyoglobin. The deconvoluted spectrum indicating a single signal.

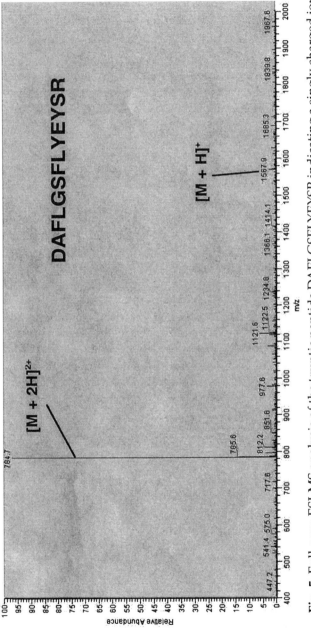

Fig. 5. Full-scan ESI-MS analysis of the tryptic peptide DAFLGSFLYEYSR indicating a singly charged ion at m/z 1567.9 and a doubly charged ion at m/z 784.7.

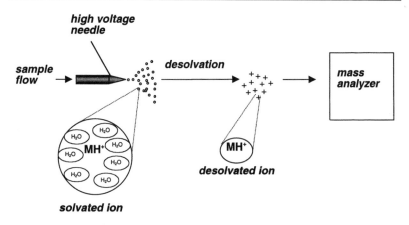

Fig. 6. Schematic representation of an ESI source.

etc.). Next, the source must separate the peptide ions from the solvent components and transfer the ions into the mass analyzer. This is accomplished in either of two ways. In some sources, the droplets pass through a heated capillary, which assists this desolvation process. In others, a curtain of nitrogen gas pass across the spray to cause desolvation. In both cases, the peptide ions pass from the source into the mass analyzer, whereas the bulk solvent from the droplets is pumped away by the vacuum system. The ions are then drawn into the mass analyzer.

6.12. Tandem Mass Analyzers

Three types of tandem mass analyzers are commonly paired with ESI sources for proteomics work. These are the triple quadrupole (commonly called the "triple quad"), the ion trap, and the quadrupole-time of flight (Q-TOF). Although these mass analyzers differ in the details of how they work, they all perform the same type of analysis. From a mixture of peptide ions generated by the ESI source, the tandem MS analyzers select a single m/z species. This ion is then subjected to *collision-induced dissociation* (CID), which induces fragmentation of the peptide into fragment ions and neutral fragments. The fragment ions are then analyzed on the basis of their m/z to produce a product ion spectrum. The information contained in this tandem or MS-MS spectrum permits the sequence of the peptide to be deduced. Moreover, the nature and sequence location of peptide modification also can be established from an MS-MS spectrum.

6.13. The Triple Quadrupole Mass Analyzer

A quadrupole mass analyzer consists of four metal rods arranged in parallel (**Fig. 7A**). Direct current and radiofrequency voltages applied to the rods create a magnetic field that causes ions to follow a corkscrew trajectory as they proceed down the axis between the rods. Depending on the voltage applied to the rods, ions of a specific m/z value will pass through the quadrupole, whereas ions of greater or lesser m/z values will fly outwards and fail to pass through the quadrupole. By sweeping the radiofrequency voltages on the rods, ions of increasing m/z values can be analyzed.

The triple quad is composed of two of these quadrupoles (Q1 and Q3, **Fig. 7B**). These are separated by a somewhat different quadrupole (q2; the lower case designation is widely accepted convention), which is governed by radiofrequency voltages only. The middle quadrupole q2 serves as a collision cell, in which collisions between ions and neutral gas atoms lead to peptide ion fragmentation. The detector is placed after Q3.

The triple quadrupole operates in two general ways. In the first, ions from the source are analyzed by rapid scanning of Q1, such that m/z values of all ions coming from the source at any given moment are recorded (**Fig. 7C**). This is referred to as "full-scan" analysis and yields signals for all the ions (e.g., singly, doubly, triply charged, etc.) coming from the source. This can be considered a "snapshot" of the peptide ions entering the source over the time interval of the scan (typically about 1 s). The other way in which the triple quad is operated is to use Q1 as a mass filter, in which the voltage settings are fixed to allow only ions of a specific m/z value to pass through (**Fig. 7D**). Those peptide ions then enter q2, where they collide with argon gas atoms and undergo fragmentation. The fragment ions thus produced are analyzed on the basis of their m/z by Q3, which scans repeatedly over a designated mass range to detect the fragment ions. This latter mode of operation is how the triple quad acquires

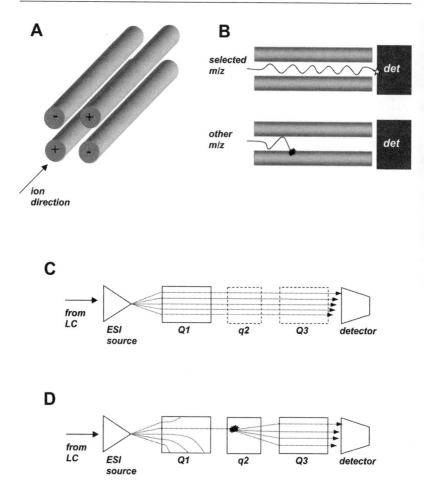

Fig. 7. Schematic representation of a triple quadrupole MS instrument.
(A) A quadrupole mass analyzer; **(B)** the trajectories of an ion of
the selected *m/z* with that of ions of other *m/z*; **(C)** operation of the
triple quad in full-scan mode; **(D)** operation of the triple quad in
MS-MS mode.

tandem MS data. The efficiency of MS-MS analysis by a triple quad depends on the properties of the peptide ions being analyzed and on instrument settings, including the pressure of Ar gas in q2 and the energy settings used for CID. In most MS-MS on triple quads, only a fraction of the precursor ions that enter q2 actually undergo fragmentation. Moreover, the fragmentation that does occur is sometimes more extensive than in an ion trap (*see* below). Thus, optimal MS-MS performance of a triple quad requires careful adjustment of instrument parameters in order to obtain an optimum degree of peptide fragmentation.

Triple quads were the original instruments used for tandem MS in proteomics studies. The accuracy of quadrupole mass analyzers allows selection of specific peptide ions (by Q1) and analysis of fragment ions from MS-MS (by Q3) to within at least ±0.5 amu of their true m/z values. This degree of mass accuracy is sufficient to allow direct interpretation of amino acid sequence from peptide MS-MS data obtained with triple quads. Moreover, these measurements of fragment ion m/z values are sufficiently accurate to permit peptide sequences by algorithms that correlate the MS-MS spectra with protein sequences obtained from databases (*see* below).

6.14. Ion-Trap Mass Analyzers

The design and operation of ion-trap mass analyzers is very different from that of triple quadrupoles. Whereas triple quads analyze and perform MS-MS on peptide ions "on the fly" as they pass through the analyzer, ion traps collect and store ions in order to perform MS-MS analyses on them. The analyzer is very simple in design. The ions from the source are directed into the ion trap, which consists of a top and bottom electrode (end caps) and a ring electrode around the middle (**Fig. 8A**). The trap itself is about the size of a grapefruit. Ions collected in the trap are maintained in orbits within the trap by a combination of DC and radiofrequency voltages. A small amount of helium is used as a "cooling gas" to help control the distribution of energies of the ions. In full-scan mode, the radiofrequency voltages on the electrodes are stepped or scanned to sequentially eject ions on the basis of their m/z values (**Fig. 8B**). This produces a spectrum representing all of the peptide ions in the trap at any given time. To monitor the ions coming from the source, the trap continuously

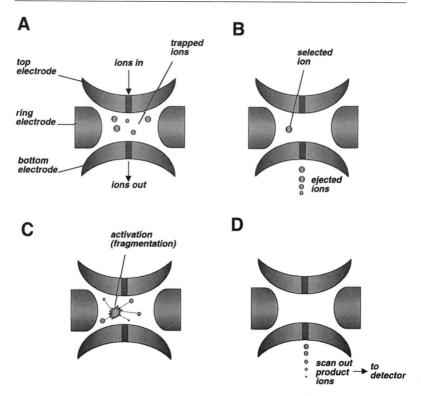

Fig. 8. Schematic representation of an ion-trap MS instrument. **(A)** Trapping of ions within the analyzer; **(B)** the sequential "scanning out" of ions of differing m/z; **(C)** collision-induced dissociation (fragmentation) of a selected ion; **(D)** depicts sequential "scanning out" of product ions derived from fragmentation of the precursor ion in (C).

repeats a cycle of: 1) filling the trap with ions, and 2) scanning the ions out according to m/z values. Thus, unlike the triple quadrupole, the ion trap produces a series of closely spaced analyses, rather than a continuous analysis. Like the triple quad, the ion trap detects multiply charged peptide ions formed by ESI, as long as their m/z values fall within the mass range limit of the analyzer.

To perform MS-MS analyses, the trap fills with ions from the source. Then a particular ion of interest is selected and the trap voltages are adjusted to eject ions of all other m/z values (**Fig. 8B**). The voltages on the trap then are quickly increased to increase the energies of the remaining ions, which results in energetic collisions of the peptide ions with the helium gas atoms in the trap and induces fragmentation of the ions (**Fig. 8C**). The fragments then are caught in the trap and scanned out in according to their m/z values (**Fig. 8D**).

A good analogy often used to describe MS analysis by ion traps is "rocks in a can." According to that analogy, we can summarize the ion trap MS-MS experiment: a handful of different-sized rocks are scooped up in a can. Then all but one are thrown out. The can is then rattled hard and the remaining rock fragments become pebbles, which then are let out one at a time and weighed.

A unique feature of traps is that fragment ions from an MS-MS experiment can themselves be retained in the trap and subjected to another round of fragmentation. Fragments from this secondary MS-MS analysis can likewise be retained and further fragmented. This type of analysis is referred to as MS^n and can yield highly detailed fragmentation information is certain cases. However, MS^n analyses are seldom used in proteomics, for two reasons. First, there is currently no way to anticipate what MS-MS-MS experiments need to be done while an analysis is underway. One does not necessarily know what ions will be formed in the MS-MS analysis of a peptide ion, so one cannot readily select a fragment for further fragmentation. Second, the total numbers of ions decrease with the number of MS cycles. After an MS-MS analysis, there frequently are not enough ions left in the trap to perform useful analyses.

There are a couple of other features that distinguish ion traps from triple quadrupoles for tandem MS analyses. The first is that fragmentation patterns generated by MS-MS of peptide ions in ion traps can differ somewhat from those produced by triple quadrupoles. Under the most commonly used operating conditions, traps tend to induce a much more complete fragmentation of the precursor ion than do quadrupoles. This means that more of the precursor ions are converted more efficiently to product ions (and thereby to sequence information) in ion traps. Indeed, the precursor ion signal usually is not seen in ion-trap MS-MS spectra, whereas it often is a prominent feature of triple quad MS-MS spectra. Although we shall consider the key features of peptide ion MS-MS spectra in Chapter 9, we can point out here that triple quads tend to induce a more diverse range of fragmentations in MS-MS than do ion traps. Most of the fragmentations produced by ion traps are those most directly useful in deducing sequence, whereas triple quad MS-MS spectra may yield additional features that can resolve ambiguities and provide additional detail. A final difference between ion traps and triple quadrupoles is the so-called "low m/z cutoff" for MS-MS in traps. Owing to the way the ion trap functions for MS-MS, it is not possible to record the masses of product ions whose m/z values are below about 25% of the m/z value of the precursor ion that was subjected to MS-MS. Thus, an ion at m/z 250 would be the lowest fragment ion that can be detected in MS-MS analysis of a m/z 1000 precursor ion. This is not usually a problem for peptide MS-MS analysis, because identities of low-mass peptide fragments can generally be deduced from the m/z values of corresponding larger fragments.

One last interesting feature to note about ion traps is that they actually are capable of very high mass resolution. However, the resolution of the trap decreases with the speed at which ions are scanned out and detected. At the scan rates typically used for full-scan and MS-MS analysis of peptides traps can adequately resolve ions that differ by at least 1 amu on the m/z scale. If the rate of scanning is slowed, traps can resolve species differing by as little as 0.05 units on the m/z scale. In automated operation, a combination of slow full scans over a limited mass range can be used to determine accurately the charge state of ions prior to MS-MS analysis. As we will see, information on the charge state of the precursor can be very helpful in determining peptide sequence from MS-MS data.

6.15. Automated Data Acquisition

Some instrument control software allows the automated switching of the triple quad or ion trap between full-scan and tandem MS modes to acquire peptide MS-MS spectra. In this approach, the instrument is set by default in full-scan mode to detect peptide ions as they emerge from the source. When peptide ions are detected, the instrument selects the most intense ion and subjects it to CID to obtain an MS-MS spectrum. The instrument then switches back to full-scan mode and selects the next most intense peptide ion and subjects it to CID. This

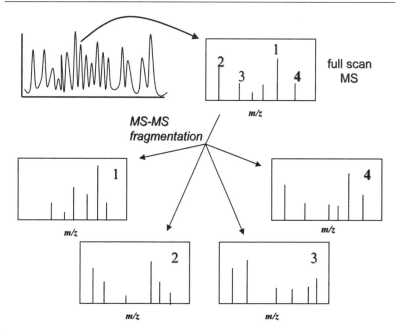

Fig. 9. Schematic representation of the automated collection of MS-MS spectra by data-dependent scanning.

switching cycle is repeated to obtain MS-MS spectra of multiple peptide ions automatically (**Fig. 9**). This automated instrument control approach is referred to as data-dependent scanning or data-dependent MS-MS and is well-suited to acquisition of large numbers of MS-MS spectra of peptides in LC-MS-MS analysis of complex peptide mixtures.

6.16. Other Mass Analyzers: Q-TOF and Fourier Transform-Ion Cyclotron Resonance MS Instruments

Two new types of mass analyzers are beginning to have an impact on analytical proteomics. Both use ESI sources. The first is the quadrupole-time of flight mass analyzer, which is commonly referred to as a Q-TOF, after the common acronyms for its two components. (It should be pointed out that the hybrid acronym "Q-TOF" is the trade name of a commercially available instrument. I use the acronym here only in the interest of brevity and clarity, not as a product endorsement.) The Q-TOF is functionally identical to a triple quad, except that the quadrupole Q3 is replaced by a TOF mass analyzer. Recent improvements in TOF technology (discussed earlier) have made these analyzers very fast and capable of very high resolution. In the Q-TOF, full-scan and MS-MS experiments are done in the same way as they are on the triple quad, except that the product ions in MS-MS are analyzed by the TOF mass analyzer rather than the quadrupole Q3. The key advantage of the Q-TOF is that the TOF is capable of much higher mass resolution that the quadrupole. Thus, very accurate mass measurements of product ions can be done. This increases the chances of obtaining accurate sequence assignments from interpretation of the MS-MS spectra. In addition, the higher resolution and mass accuracy of the TOF yield data that may be more effectively used in software-assisted data interpretation.

The Fourier transform ion cyclotron resonance MS (known as FT-ICR or most commonly, FT-MS) is somewhat analogous to an ion trap. However, the mass analyzer employs a powerful magnetic field (typically 3–7 Tesla) and Fourier transform algorithm to detect all ions in the trap simultaneously. These instruments can be operated with ESI sources and can achieve spectacular resolution even for very complex peptide mixtures. FT-MS instruments are potentially very powerful tools for analytical proteomics. However, they are very expensive and somewhat temperamental instruments and these factors have limited their impact on proteomics.

Suggested Reading

Jonscher, K. R. and Yates, J. R. (1997) The quadrupole ion trap mass spectrometer: a small solution to a big challenge. *Anal. Biochem.* **244,** 1–15.

Siuzdak, G. (1996) *Mass Spectrometry for Biotechnology.* Academic Press, San Diego.

Stahl, D. C., Swiderek, K. M., Davis, M. T., and Lee, T. D. (1995) Data-controlled automation of liquid chromatography/tandem mass spectrometry analysis of peptide mixtures. *J. Am. Soc. Mass Spectrom.* **7,** 532–540.

Yates, J. R. (1998) Mass spectrometry and the age of the proteome. *J. Mass. Spectrom.* **33,** 1–19.

7 Protein Identification by Peptide Mass Fingerprinting

7.1. What is Peptide Mass Fingerprinting?

Peptide mass fingerprinting is a protein identification technique in which MS is used to measure the masses of proteolytic peptide fragments. The protein then is identified by matching the measured peptide masses to corresponding peptide masses from protein or nucleotide sequence databases. Peptide mass fingerprinting works well for analytical proteomics because it combines a conceptually simple approach with robust, high-throughput instrumentation (typically MALDI-TOF MS). As with other MS-based analytical proteomics techniques, the quality of the protein identifications made depend on the quality of both the MS data, the accuracy of the databases, and the power of the search algorithms and software used. In the remainder of this chapter, we will consider peptide mass fingerprinting in greater detail. We will describe how peptide mass measurements can be used to identify proteins and finally how algorithms and software can automate the identification process.

7.2. Peptide Mass Fingerprinting: Overview

Imagine for a moment that we could take the entire proteome of an organism and cleave it to a collection of tryptic peptides. Remember, trypsin cleaves proteins very selectively by cutting at lysine and arginine residues (except those next to prolines). Thus, tryptic digestion of each protein yields a specific number of peptides of specific

From: *Introduction to Proteomics: Tools for the New Biology*
By: D. C. Liebler © Humana Press, Inc., Totowa, NJ

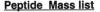

Peptide Mass list

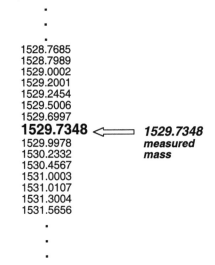

.
.
.
1528.7685
1528.7989
1529.0002
1529.2001
1529.2454
1529.5006
1529.6997
1529.7348 ⟸ *1529.7348*
1529.9978   *measured*
1530.2332   *mass*
1530.4567
1531.0003
1531.0107
1531.3004
1531.5656
.
.
.

Fig. 1. Matching of a peptide *m/z* value against a peptide ion mass list generated from a protein-sequence database.

length, sequence, and most importantly, of specific mass. As long as each peptide in the collection were associated with its protein of origin and amino acid sequence position, all of the information in the proteome would be maintained. Of course, we do not have to do this experimentally. We can use a computer to generate this list of peptides by performing a virtual digestion of all the proteins in a database. We also can do this with nucleotide sequence information by converting it to protein sequence information and then digesting. In principle, a complete genome sequence, properly annotated, can yield a complete list of proteins and, consequently, of tryptic peptides.

This super-list of peptides now becomes a valuable reference tool. One could rank these tryptic peptides from lowest mass to highest. An inspection of this list would reveal that some of the peptides over about six amino acids in length (about 700 Da) would have unique masses.

Now, let's imagine that we have in hand some unknown protein from that organism and we wish to identify it. We start by digesting the protein with trypsin to generate tryptic peptides. Each peptide we get from this digestion has a mass. Let's assume that we can know the exact mass of each of our tryptic peptide digestion products. If we were to take one of the tryptic peptide masses and compare it to the entries on the list, we would find a peptide on the list with exactly the same mass (**Fig. 1**). If the measured mass was unique in the list of all peptide masses, we would be almost certain that the peptides are identical. Because we know the sequence location and origin of the peptide match in the list, we can be fairly sure that our tryptic peptide came from that same protein. We can then take a second tryptic peptide from our unknown protein and match it to the list in the same way. Again, a match would indicate which peptide and parent protein corresponded to our unknown. Several matches between our tryptic peptides and tryptic peptide masses all from the same protein in the list would confirm the identity of our unknown. Even if multiple entries in the peptide mass list matched one of our unknown tryptic peptides, a consistent set of "hits" on peptides all derived from the same protein in the list would confirm our assignment. Thus, as long as we can match peptide masses to a good list, we can identify unknowns simply by measuring the masses of their tryptic peptides. This is the essence of protein identification by peptide mass fingerprinting.

Of course, this was a highly idealized example. We were blessed with perfect mass measurements of our unknown tryptic peptides and a perfect list of all possible tryptic peptides from the proteins in our target organism. Successful application of peptide mass fingerprinting depends on how close we can come to perfection in the real world. Practically speaking, successful protein identification by peptide mass fingerprinting requires two things. First, one must be able to make accurate measurements of peptide masses. Second, one must have accurate databases of protein sequence to work with.

7.3. Peptide Mass Fingerprinting: Analytical Approach

The approach to peptide mass fingerprinting is reasonably simple. A protein sample is treated with a specific protease (most commonly trypsin), which cleaves the protein in a predictable way. We do not need to use trypsin, of course. There are a number of other proteases and even chemical reagents that can specifically cleave proteins to

Table 1
Effect of Mass Accuracy and Mass Tolerance on Peptide
Mass Fingerprinting Search Result[a]

Search m/z	Mass tolerance (Da)	# Hits
1529	1	478
1529.7	0.1	164
1529.73	0.01	25
1529.734	0.001	4
1529.7348	0.0001	2

[a]Searches were done with the MS-FIT program at http://
prospector.ucsf.edu/

peptides. However, the key is generating specific cleavages. This is
because we have to subject our database of protein sequence to the
same cleavages to generate a peptide mass list to match against. The
peptides then are analyzed by MS to obtain mass measurements.
Remember, the instruments actually measure m/z values, which can
be converted to masses. In principle, any MS instrument can be used
to measure peptide m/z values. However, reliable and unambiguous
protein identification by peptide mass fingerprinting requires highly
accurate mass measurements. The importance of this point is easy to
illustrate with a real peptide.

Tryptic digestion of human hemoglobin alpha chain yields 14 tryptic
peptides, of which the peptide VGAHAGEYGAEALER has an exact
monoisotopic mass of 1528.7348 Da. Thus, the singly charged ion of
this peptide has an m/z value of 1529.7348. The results of searching this
peptide against all mouse and human proteins in the SWISS-PROT
database are illustrated in **Table 1**.

If we were able to measure only to the nearest whole m/z value
(i.e., a measured m/z of 1529) with a mass tolerance of 1 Da (i.e., the
measured mass can be within ±1 Da of the true value), there are
478 matches. In other words, 478 tryptic peptides from mouse and
human proteins are within ±1 Da of 1529. However, if we can make
more accurate m/z measurements of the peptide ion and use more
stringent mass tolerances, we can narrow the match eventually to
two peptides. Interestingly, these are VGAHAGEYGAEALER from
human hemoglobin alpha and IGGHGAEYGAEALER from mouse

Table 2
Protein Matches for Peptide Mass Fingerprinting
of m/z 1529.73 Peptide

Peptide sequence	Identification	Matched m/z (difference) from search mass
IGGHGAEYGAEALER	Mouse Hb alpha	1529.7348 (−0.0048)
VGAHAGEYGAEALER	Human Hb alpha	1529.7348 (−0.0048)
MGTGWEGMYRTLK	Mouse lens epithelial cell protein LEP503	1529.7245 (0.0055)
MADEEKLPPGWEK	Human PIN1-like protein	1529.7310 (−0.0010)
DTQTSITDSSAIYK	Mouse signal recognition particle receptor beta subunit	1529.7335 (−0.0035)
NDSSPNPVYQPPSK	Mouse peroxisome assembly factor-1	1529.7236 (0.0064)
MNLSLNDAYDFVK	Human dual specificity protein phosphatase 7	1529.7310 (0.0010)

hemoglobin alpha. Both have m/z values of 1529.7348, even though they differ by four amino acid substitutions.

The key point here is that more accurate m/z measurements provide more useful data for peptide mass fingerprinting. For this approach to work the MS instrumentation used must be able to measure peptide masses to within 0.05 Da of the actual values. Modern MALDI-TOF instruments with delayed extraction and reflectron analyzers are capable of this and are most widely used for this purpose. However, a search with the single m/z value 1529.73 and a mass tolerance of ±0.01 Da still yielded 25 hits (**Table 1**). The proteins corresponding to some of these are listed in **Table 2**.

All of the matches are well within the specified mass tolerance of 0.01 Da. By that criterion, any of these matches could be our protein. So how do we identify the right protein from these very similar matches?

The answer is that accurate protein identifications usually require *multiple* peptide matches. In the example in **Table 1**, even the best possible mass match was unable to tell us whether the peptide we

Table 3
Effects of Multiple Peptide Masses on Protein
Identification by Peptide Mass Fingerprinting[a]

Search m/z[b]	Mass tolerance	# Hits
1529.73	0.1	204
1529.73 1252.70	0.1	7
1529.73 1252.70 1833.88	0.1	1

[a]Searches were done with the MS-FIT program at http://prospector.ucsf.edu/

[b]The actual peptide m/z values are 1529.7348 (VGAHA GEYGAEALER), 1252.7074 (FLASVSTVLTSK) and 1833.8845 (TYFPHFDLSHGSAQVK).

analyzed was from human or mouse hemoglobin. However, any real tryptic digestion of the protein sample would have yielded multiple peptides and given us multiple m/z values to search against the database. The benefit of increasing the number of peptide m/z values searched is illustrated in **Table 3**.

Searches with one or two peptide m/z values from human hemoglobin alpha yielded multiple hits. However, a search with three peptide m/z values of the 14 possible human hemoglobin alpha tryptic peptides yielded a single hit for the correct protein.

7.4. Peptide Mass Fingerprinting: Complications

We used very simple examples earlier to illustrate the concepts of protein identification by peptide mass fingerprinting. With m/z measurements from two or three peptides, identification of their protein precursor as human hemoglobin alpha was relatively straightforward. Of course, we "cheated" a little by making the peptide masses both correct and exact to 0.01 Da or better. The examples demonstrated that more precise, accurate peptide mass measurements and good mass measurements on multiple peptides greatly increased the accuracy of identification. With data from only two or three peptides, one could envision doing peptide mass fingerprinting "by hand" with success.

However, several factors complicate peptide mass fingerprinting in the real world. First, real MS data on peptides are not as perfect as in the previous examples. Although most modern MALDI-TOF instruments equipped with reflectrons or delayed extraction are capable of measuring the m/z values of peptide ions to within 0.005 unit or better, errors nevertheless are inevitable. Second, there are frequently a lot of signals in MALDI-TOF spectra of real samples and many are from more than one protein. Consider that most spots on 2D gels contain 2–3 proteins, that a typical 50 kDa protein may give rise to 25–40 tryptic peptides, and that other contaminants in the sample (e.g., human keratin from careless sample handling). These factors combine to produce spectra that are complex and represent peptides from multiple proteins. Finally, there is always a possibility that some database matches are owing to chance alone, rather than actual identity. The possibility of false-positive matches is greater for larger proteins, mainly because they yield more tryptic peptides than do smaller proteins.

7.5 Software Tools for Peptide Mass Fingerprinting: Finding the Matches

Although the volume of data and the calculations involved may seem overwhelming, we can look to data-reduction algorithms and software for help. There are a number of software tools available to facilitate protein identification by peptide mass fingerprinting. Several are listed later in this chapter. What follows is a generic description of what these programs do.

Typically, the user begins by selecting the database(s) to be searched. Both protein and/or gene sequence databases may be specified (gene sequences are translated if the latter is selected). An excellent, widely used protein sequence database is the SWISS-PROT database. Other widely used protein sequence databases are the OWL and NCBInr databases. The user then can provide information about the origin of the sample to limit the search to relevant organisms. For example, a sample from mouse proteins can be searched against all organisms, against mammalian sequences, against rodents, or most specifically, against mouse sequences. Specificity is advantageous because it can limit the number of comparisons to be made with the data and because it can limit the number "false" hits in other organisms. In addition to these features, the user may also enter a molecular-weight range for proteins to be searched. This again limits the number of comparisons to be made.

Next, the user can indicate the enzyme used to cleave the proteins (e.g., trypsin) and specify the possible numbers of "missed cleavages." These missed cleavages result from incomplete digestion by the enzyme. The matching algorithms thus can generate entries for such peptides, in case they are present in the sample. Finally, the user can specify a number of standard modifications to peptides that can be considered in the matching algorithm. For example, tryptic-digestion protocols usually involve a reduction and alkylation of cysteine thiols with iodoacetamide or iodoacetate, which changes the masses of the cysteine residues within peptides. In addition, free cysteine thiols may undergo modification with acrylamide during SDS-PAGE. The user can also specify common modifications such as phosphorylation, sulfation, glycosylation, and N-terminal modifications. All these user-defined modifications allow the program to generate mass matches for both modified and unmodified versions of the peptides in a data-base. MS data for both modified and unmodified versions of a particular peptide can thus be matched to a database entry. The user then can enter the measured m/z values from the MS data or specify an MS datafile to be evaluated automatically. Finally, the user can enter a desired mass tolerance to control how closely the matches between MS m/z values and calculated m/z values must correspond to be "hits."

Once the user clicks "Go," the software begins by prefiltering the database to be used. For example, if mouse was specified as the species to be searched, all nonmouse entries are excluded. If a protein mass range of 2,000–100,000 was selected, all proteins with masses outside this range are excluded. Then the remaining sequences in the databases are subjected to a virtual digestion with the enzyme specified. If missed cleavages are allowed, the list of peptides will include those resulting from incomplete digestion. Versions of the peptides bearing the user-specified modifications are also generated. Finally, the entire list of peptides is ranked by mass (or m/z values) and each m/z signal in each spectrum is then compared to this list. All matches within the user-specified mass tolerances are recorded as "hits" and used for calculation of scores and identification of corresponding proteins.

7.6. Software Tools for Peptide Mass Fingerprinting: Scoring the Results

In MALDI-TOF spectra from real samples, there are typically dozens of m/z signals. Peptide mass fingerprinting software can usually match just about all of these to some entry in a database. However, given errors in m/z measurement, frequent sample contamination, and the presence of unanticipated posttranslational modifications, not all of the matches will point to the same proteins. So how do we score the hits to determine which protein best matches the data?

The simplest approach is to assign the highest score to proteins whose predicted tryptic peptides match the greatest number of m/z signals in the MS data. If we search only one m/z value, then several proteins could be equally good matches. However, as we search a greater number of m/z values, more matches correspond to a particular protein and lead to a greater score for that protein vs others. This fairly simple approach works reasonably well with very good MS data. However, it tends to assign higher scores to larger proteins. As noted earlier, larger proteins yield more tryptic peptides, so the chances of a match to one of these is greater for larger proteins than for smaller proteins.

To address these problems, several of the available peptide mass fingerprinting programs use more sophisticated scoring algorithms. These algorithms correct for scoring bias due to protein size, in which larger proteins give rise to greater numbers of peptides. They also correct for the tendency of smaller peptides in databases to have a greater number of matches with searched m/z values. Finally, some of these algorithms also apply probability-based statistics to better define the significance of protein identifications. At the time of this writing, the principal tools available for peptide mass fingerprinting can be grouped into three categories:

- First-generation freeware and subscription software tools that assign scores based on the number of m/z values in a spectrum that match database values within a given mass tolerance. These programs include PepSea (http://www.protana.com) and Pept Ident/MultIdent (http://www.expasy.ch/tools/peptident.html).

- Second-generation freeware and subscription software tools that employ scoring algorithms that take into account the effects of protein size and peptide length on the probabilities of matching. These include MOWSE (http://srs.hgmp.mrc.ac.uk/cgi-bin/mowse) and MS-Fit (http://prospector.ucsf.edu/).
- Third-generation software that employs more extensive probability-based scoring to provide a statistical basis for scores and also to estimate the probabilities that matches may reflect random events, rather than true identities. These programs include ProFound (http://prowl.rockefeller.edu/cgi-bin/Pro Found) and Mascot (http://www.matrixscience.com/).

7.7. Peptide Mass Fingerprinting: Assessment and Outlook

The peptide mass fingerprinting approach to protein identification has much to recommend it. First, it is the closest thing to "high-throughput" in proteomics. With the aid of automation in sample preparation, MS analysis, and data reduction, hundreds of protein identifications can be done per day with a single system. The instrumentation (typically MALDI-TOF) is user-friendly, robust, and sensitive. The rapid evolution of protein and nucleotide sequence databases provides an ever more reliable platform for database-search algorithms. Finally, improvements in search algorithms and the application of sophisticated statistical methods has improved the reliability of protein assignments.

However, there remain several limitations to peptide mass fingerprinting. First, both the lack of complete and accurately annotated genome- and protein-sequence databases for humans and many other widely studied species limits the quality of matches that can be achieved, even with excellent MS data and software. This situation surely will improve, but remains a significant limitation in the near term. Second, the greater number of highly homologous proteins in higher organisms complicates the problem of distinguishing between closely related proteins, whose peptide maps are highly similar. Peptide mass fingerprinting may be a slam-dunk in yeast, but it is much trickier in mice and humans. Third, peptide mass fingerprinting is primarily a protein identification technique. As we shall see later, in proteomics applications beyond identification, information about peptide sequence and sites of peptide modification are essential. We cannot deduce these things from peptide mass measurements.

Despite these concerns, peptide mass fingerprinting is an essential capability of any serious proteomics laboratory. Many of the limitations of MALDI-TOF-based peptide mass fingerprinting can be overcome by the use of ESI-tandem MS, which we will examine in the next two chapters.

Suggested Reading

Fenyo, D. (2000) Identifying the proteome: software tools. *Curr. Opin. Biotechnol.* **11**, 391–395.

Gras, R., Muller, M., Gasteiger, E., Gay, S., Binz, P. A., Bienvenut, W., et al. (1999) Improving protein identification from peptide mass fingerprinting through a parameterized multi-level scoring algorithm and an optimized peak detection. *Electrophoresis* **20**, 3535–3550.

Jensen, O. N., Podtelejnikov, A. V., and Mann, M. (1997) Identification of the components of simple protein mixtures by high-accuracy peptide mass mapping and database searching. *Anal. Chem.* **69**, 4741–4750.

8 Peptide Sequence Analysis by Tandem Mass Spectrometry

8.1. What's in a Pattern?

In the last chapter, we considered protein identification with an m/z measurement of the tryptic peptide VGAHAGEYGAEALER from human hemoglobin alpha. When we searched a human/mouse protein sequence database, we found two "perfect" hits for this peptide, both of which had m/z 1529.7384 for the $[M+H]^+$ ion. Both corresponded to hemoglobin alpha peptides that are highly conserved between mice and men:

The human:	VGAHAGEYGAEALER
The mouse:	IGGHGAEYGAEALER

Nevertheless, a quick glance at the two sequences together immediately registers that "IGG" and "VGA" are different. A second, more careful look shows that "HGA" and "HAG", are close, but different. What we perceive is a *pattern* that distinguishes two species that are identical in one way (mass), yet are obviously different. In this chapter, we will consider how tandem MS analysis induces peptide fragmentation, how fragmentation generates product ions in MS-MS spectra, and how we can determine peptide sequence from fragmentation patterns in MS-MS spectra.

8.2. What's in a Peptide Sequence?

The use of the aforementioned letters illustrates differences in pattern and structure between two peptides of identical mass. However,

From: *Introduction to Proteomics: Tools for the New Biology*
By: D. C. Liebler © Humana Press, Inc., Totowa, NJ

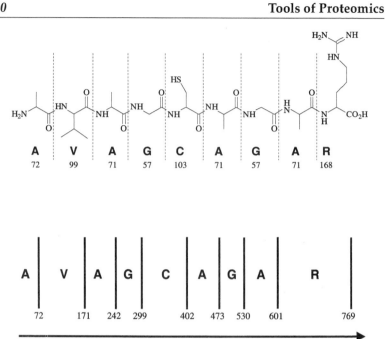

cumulative mass

Fig. 1. Representation of the peptide AVAGCAGAR as a construct of amino acid "building blocks" of different masses.

MS instruments measure m/z values for peptides and their fragments and thus reduce these structures to patterns of numbers. Understanding the number pattern scheme for peptide structure is essential to understanding what information is contained in tandem MS spectra. Let's consider the peptide AVAGCAGAR, which will serve as our model to illustrate key concepts of tandem MS fragmentation. The primary structure of this peptide is depicted in **Fig. 1**, which depicts the sequence in a linear fashion. Remember that peptides are synthesized by end-to-end condensation of amino acids with loss of water to form peptide bonds. The amino acid residues of the AVAGCAGAR peptide in **Fig. 1** are denoted by the dotted lines, which denote the amino acid residues. Each residue has an amide NH group at one end, a C = O group at the other, and an alpha carbon with one proton in the middle.

Table 1
Average Residue Masses of Amino Acids

Amino acid	One-letter code	Average residue mass
Glycine	G	57.05
Alanine	A	71.08
Serine	S	87.08
Proline	P	97.12
Valine	V	99.13
Threonine	T	101.11
Cysteine	C	103.14
Leucine	L	113.16
Isoleucine	I	113.16
Asparagine	N	114.10
Aspartic acid	D	115.09
Lysine	K	128.17
Glutamine	Q	128.13
Glutamic acid	E	129.12
Methionine	M	131.19
Histidine	H	137.14
Phenylalanine	F	147.18
Arginine	R	156.19
Tyrosine	Y	163.18
Tryptophan	W	186.21

The side chains that give each amino acid its special chemistry are attached to the alpha carbon. The amino acid units that contain these elements are referred to as residues and **Table 1** lists the identities and residue masses for the common amino acids.

With such a table to convert the amino acid letter names to amino acid residue masses, we can represent a series of amino acids as a series of numbers, which correspond to the masses of its amino acid residues. To complete the structure, we must add an extra proton (1 amu) to the N-terminal residue and an extra OH (17 amu) to the C-terminal amino acid. We now can represent the AVAGCAGAR peptide as a cumulative number series as shown in the lower part of **Fig. 1**. It is this number series that most closely represents how the MS instrument sees this peptide and its sequence.

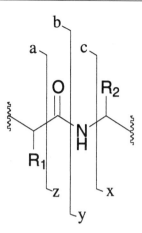

Fig. 2. Schematic representation of nomenclature for fragmentation of peptide ions.

8.3. Peptide Ion Fragmentation in MS-MS

When peptide ions collide with neutral gas atoms in the collision cell of a triple quad or a Q-TOF or in an ion trap, the kinetic energy they absorb induces fragmentation. Although many bonds in peptides could possibly undergo fragmentation, the most significant cleavages are along the peptide backbone (**Fig. 2**). A widely accepted nomenclature is used to describe peptide ion fragmentation. In the most commonly observed cleavage, the bond between the carbonyl oxygen and the amide nitrogen is cleaved to form a "y-ion" and a "b-ion." A y-ion is a fragment in which the positive charge is retained on the C-terminus of the original peptide ion; a b-ion is a fragment in which the charge is retained on the N-terminal portion of the original peptide ion. Doubly charged ions are most likely to have charges at the opposite ends of the molecule. When these peptide ions fragment, both a b-ion and the corresponding y-ion are formed. When singly charged ions fragment, either a b-ion or a y-ion is formed. The other half of the peptide is lost as a neutral fragment. Obviously, one gets twice as much information from fragmentation of doubly charged as opposed to singly charged ions.

Figure 2 also depicts other cleavages of the peptide backbone. The a-, b-, x-, and z-ions shown are observed occasionally in MS-MS spectra obtained on ion traps, triple quads, and Q-TOF instruments. However, their appearance is unusual, as these fragmentations require more energy than the cleavages that yield b- and y-ions. (They are observed with greater frequency in tandem MS analyses on magnetic sector instruments, which utilize greater energies for collision-induced dissociation of peptide ions.)

8.4. The MS-MS Spectrum

To better understand how b- and y-ion fragmentations yield a signature pattern, it is helpful to consider the spectrum of a peptide. The predicted b- and y-ion fragmentations for the model peptide AVAGCAGAR are depicted in **Fig. 3**. The actual MS-MS spectrum of the doubly charged ion of AVAGCAGAR is shown in **Fig. 4**. In looking at the peptide ion from the N-terminus (i.e., the left), cleavages yield an ascending series of fragment ion m/z values (the b-series) and a complementary descending series (the y-series). The b_4- and y_5-ion fragments generated by cleavage of the G-C bond are also depicted. Each bears a single charge. The sites of protonation in the depicted fragments are slightly different than in the intact precursor. These structures represent species conventionally agreed as likely to be present in the gas phase upon collision-induced dissociation. However, multiple forms of the ions with protonation at different sites along the chains all exist together. Proton migration to the peptide amide nitrogens in the doubly charged precursor is thought to help drive cleavage of adjacent peptide bonds in collision-induced dissociation.

The most important thing about the b- and y-ion series in the MS-MS spectrum is that they indicate the sequence of the peptide. Let's start by considering just the y-ion series. In this example, the gap between the ions labeled y_7 and y_6 is 71 amu, which corresponds to the residue mass of an alanine. The gap between the y_6 and y_5 ions is 57, which corresponds to a glycine. The gap between y_5 and y_4 is 103, which corresponds to cysteine. Just this short segment of the y-ion series establishes the presence of an "AGC" motif in the peptide. The complete y-ion series (y_8 through y_1) indicates the "VAGCAGAR" motif.

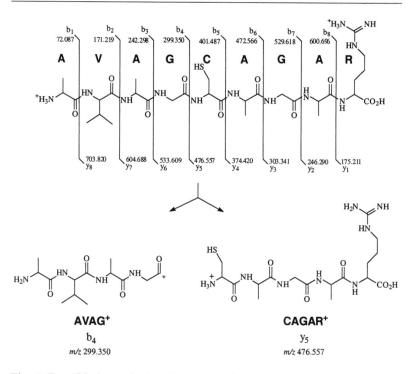

Fig. 3. Possible b- and y-ion fragments for the peptide AVAGCAGAR. Structures of the b_4 and y_5 ions from cleavage between the glycine and cysteine residues are depicted.

The b-ion series complements the y-ion series. The gap between the b_7 and b_6 ions is 57, which corresponds to glycine. The gap between b_6 and b_5 is 71, which corresponds to alanine. The complete b-ion series (b_8 through b_1) corresponds to the "AVAGCAGA" motif. Thus, the y- and b-ion series describe the same amino acid sequence in two different directions. Accordingly, the assignment of b- and y-ions in the MS-MS spectrum (**Fig. 4**) of the AVAGACAGAR doubly charged ion provides definitive confirmation of sequence.

Of course, we began this example knowing the sequence of the peptide. In the real world, we usually do not know the sequence of the peptide, so we obtain an MS-MS spectrum. We then must sit down with the spectrum, a calculator, and table of residual amino acid

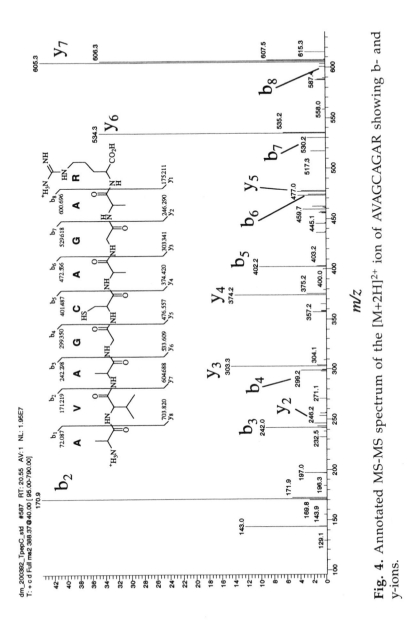

Fig. 4. Annotated MS-MS spectrum of the $[M+2H]^{2+}$ ion of AVAGCAGAR showing b- and y-ions.

masses (e.g., **Table 1**) and identify the b- and y-ions in the spectrum in order to interpret the sequence of the peptide. This is called *de novo* sequence interpretation. Depending on one's level of experience and the quality of data, a spectrum can be interpreted in anywhere from 15 min to several hours. This is fine, except when we consider that a single LC tandem MS analysis can generate hundreds or thousands of MS-MS spectra, all of which may represent different peptide sequences. Clearly, manual *de novo* sequence interpretation of so many spectra cannot realistically keep up with the volume of data we can generate.

To address this need, data-reduction algorithms and software tools have been developed to compare MS-MS data to peptide sequences in databases to identify the proteins from which the peptides were derived. These programs include Sequest and several other similar tools, which will be described in more detail below. Before we discuss these, it is important to consider other features of MS-MS spectra that can be informative, as well as problems and anomalies commonly encountered in MS-MS analysis of peptides.

8.5. Problems, Peculiarities, and Proline

The MS-MS spectrum for the AVAGCAGAR peptide in **Fig. 4** is not very different from MS-MS spectra commonly encountered in LC-tandem MS analyses of peptides. However, not all spectra are this pretty. Of course, at the limits of instrument sensitivity, the spectra can be incomplete and hard to interpret. However, even when the amount of peptide being analyzed is well above the detection limit, several things can prevent the instrument from generating a "perfect" MS-MS spectrum with a complete b- and y-ion series. These include: 1) differences in tendencies of different peptide bonds to fragment, 2) unique fragmentation characteristics of certain amino acids, and 3) the damping effect of proline on peptide ion fragmentation.

The factors that control how easily different peptide bonds are not yet entirely understood. However, fragmentation does depend on how easily the protons in the protonated peptide ions can migrate to various in-chain peptide amide nitrogens. Sites that are most easily protonated are most easily cleaved. There also appears to be a role for stabilizing positive charges by acidic amino acid side chains. Thus, cleavages adjacent to glutamate or aspartate residues often give rise to intense fragment ions. In many peptide MS-MS spectra, the most intense ions are those arising from cleavages near the middle of the peptide. Remember, when peptide ions gain energy from collisions, the energy of fragmentation is parceled out among various competing pathways. Very facile cleavages can thus diminish the contributions of others and some fragment ions will then be weak or absent.

The fragmentation patterns of tryptic peptide ions are particularly important because so much of proteomics relies on MS analysis of tryptic protein digests. As noted earlier, tryptic peptides easily generate doubly charged ions because they have lysine or arginine residues at the C-terminus. In MS-MS spectra of tryptic peptides, the y-ion series usually is more intense than the b-ion series. This is because of the ability of the basic side chains in lysine and arginine residues to retain positive charge at the C-terminus of peptide fragments. It is also worth noting in this context that some cleavages of doubly charged peptide ions yield a doubly charged product ion and a neutral fragment. Thus, some product ions in MS-MS spectra may be from doubly charged fragments, rather than from singly charged fragments. When these occur, they usually are infrequent. However, they can sometimes confound interpretation of spectra.

Some amino acid side chains undergo cleavages that yield characteristic fragmentations that do not involve the peptide backbone. For example, serine and threonine residues easily eliminate water from their side chains, which contain hydroxyl groups. The ions generated from water loss are sometimes more intense than the ions for the intact serine- or threonine-containing fragments. An analogous loss of phosphoric acid (H_3PO_4) occurs from phosphoserine and phosphothreonine residues. The ions formed from these losses can often dominate MS-MS spectra and are frequently reliable indicators of phosphopeptides. Other characteristic side chain losses include loss of H_2S from cysteine and loss of ammonia from glutamine and asparagine.

A final contributor to ambiguity in peptide fragmentation is the occurrence of proline residues. As noted in Chapter 5, proline prevents tryptic cleavage when located on the C-terminal side of either a lysine or arginine. In addition to this effect on digestion, proline can affect MS-MS fragmentation. Proline peptide bonds are relatively resistant to fragmentation. This is owing to the unique structure of this amino acid, which has a cyclic side chain attached at both the alpha carbon and the secondary amine. In a peptide chain, the proline nitrogen does not have an available site for protonation and cleavage thus is greatly suppressed. The effect of this is missing b- or y-ions where cleavages about proline residues fail to occur.

8.6. The Definitive Approach

Tandem MS has now become the definitive approach to determination of peptide sequences. Although Edman degradation had served for many years as the standard method, there are limits to its usefulness. First, Edman degradation cannot be used to analyze peptides whose amine terminus is modified (the Edman reagent will not react with N-terminally-modified peptides). Tandem MS not only can be used to analyze N-terminally modified peptides, it can also reveal the nature of the modifications. Second, although Edman degradation can be applied to mapping some posttranslational modifications (e.g., phosphorylation) it is considerably less versatile for this purpose than mass spectrometry. This is because Edman analysis involves sequential chemical cleavage of the N-terminal residue from a peptide and identification of the cleaved derivative by chromatography. Without standards for many possible modified amino acids, Edman cannot provide definitive identification of the modified amino acids. One must also consider that some modifications may interfere with the reaction between the Edman reagents and the modified peptide.

We can now consider tandem MS the state-of-the-art approach to peptide-sequence analysis. Of course, identification of peptide sequences allows us to identify proteins by comparing the sequences to protein sequences in databases. However, there is a practical problem with doing this. The interpretation of sequence from tandem MS data can be labor-intensive and slow. The next chapter describes new tools that have been developed to overcome this problem and make tandem MS data practically useful for high-throughput protein identification.

Suggested Reading

Roepstorff, P. and Fohlman, J. (1984) Proposal for a common nomenclature for sequence ions in mass spectra of peptides. *Biomed. Mass Spectrom.* **11,** 601–601.

Yates, J. R. (1998) Mass spectrometry and the age of the proteome. *J. Mass. Spectrom.* **33,** 1–19.

9 Protein Identification with Tandem Mass Spectrometry Data

9.1. Applying ESI Tandem MS to Protein Identification

There are two ways to identify proteins from peptide MS-MS spectra. The first is *de novo* interpretation of the spectrum to obtain a peptide sequence followed by BLAST searching of the sequence against a sequence database to identify the protein. This is a perfectly reasonable approach—as long as there are only a few spectra to deal with. Manual *de novo* interpretation of an individual MS-MS spectrum takes between half an hour and a couple of days, depending on the complexity of the spectrum and the experience of the analyst. As noted earlier, some spectra do not contain complete b- or y-ion series and thus it may not be possible to unambiguously interpret a peptide sequence from these spectra. The analyst then must guess at sequence where the spectral clues fall short. Of course, accurate *de novo* interpretation of MS-MS spectra requires skill and experience. Nevertheless, we could easily use this approach to assign the sequences of several peptides in a sample and identify the precursor protein by BLAST searching within a day or two. This could be perfectly acceptable, for example, to identify one or two proteins from bands on an SDS gel.

From: *Introduction to Proteomics: Tools for the New Biology*
By: D. C. Liebler © Humana Press, Inc., Totowa, NJ

Unfortunately, the emerging field of proteomics relies on identification of large numbers of proteins from MS-MS spectra. Clearly, the *de novo* sequencing/BLAST searching approach will be too slow for large-scale protein identification. The "slow step" in this case is the manual inspection of MS-MS spectra to determine sequence. This is where the second approach to protein identification with MS-MS data comes into play.

The second approach to protein identification bypasses the "slow step" (manual *de novo* sequence interpretation). In this approach, algorithms are applied to directly correlate MS-MS spectral data with peptide sequences in databases without actually interpreting each MS-MS spectrum individually. How such tools work will be described below. However, it is important to appreciate how well this second approach fits with the emerging database resources brought about by genome sequencing. If we accept that an algorithm can identify proteins by matching peptide MS-MS spectra to database sequences, the only limitations to such an approach are the quality of the MS-MS spectra and the completeness and accuracy of the databases.

If we obtain an MS-MS spectrum of a peptide whose sequence exists in a database, the right algorithm should be able to make the match. The algorithms discussed below can match MS-MS data to protein sequences or to nucleotide (e.g., genome or EST) sequences that are translated to protein sequences. If the sequence of the analyzed peptide does not exist in the database, a correct match cannot be made. However, progress in genome sequencing of humans and other organisms makes such databases more accurate and complete virtually every day. Indeed, in the near future, complete protein-sequence databases for all genes in organisms with sequenced genomes will be available. This emerging body of database information gives analytical proteomics approaches ever-growing power and reliability.

9.2. Algorithms and Software Tools for Identifying Proteins from ESI Tandem MS Data: Sequest

The first algorithm/program to identify proteins by matching MS-MS data to database sequences is Sequest, which was introduced by John Yates and Jimmy Eng in 1995. Several similar software tools have been introduced and these will be discussed below. However, Sequest will be described in greatest detail as representative of this class of tools. The value of programs such as Sequest is that they provide a relatively rapid assignment of MS-MS spectra to specific peptide sequences in databases. This allows fast reduction of large volumes of LC-MS-MS data in proteomics analyses. However, it is important to emphasize that Sequest and similar programs do not actually perform *de novo* interpretation of the spectra *per se*. Consequently, the output of these programs depends on the quality of the MS-MS data obtained and the completeness and accuracy of the database used.

Here's how Sequest works. When the MS instrument obtains an MS-MS scan, it not only records the MS-MS scan itself, but also the m/z value of the precursor ion. This information is stored together with the scan data. After the analysis is complete, the user sits at the computer and opens the Sequest program. The user then selects the datafile containing the MS-MS scans to be analyzed. The user can tell Sequest what enzyme (e.g., trypsin) was used to digest the protein sample and also specifies whether singly or doubly charged ions were subjected to MS-MS. Finally, the user selects a database against which the MS-MS data are to be compared.

Once the program starts, all of the proteins in the database are subjected to a virtual digestion with the enzyme specified by the user (e.g., trypsin). This generates a master list of possible peptides for comparison to the MS-MS scans. Then each MS-MS scan is analyzed as follows (**Fig. 1**):

- The precursor m/z for each MS-MS scan is used to select peptides from the database with the same mass (within a defined mass tolerance). If no digestion enzyme was specified, the program simply selects all possible peptide sequences that correspond to the mass of the peptide ion analyzed in that MS-MS scan.
- Theoretical MS-MS spectra are generated from each of the selected peptides.
- The MS-MS spectrum being analyzed is compared with each of the theoretical MS-MS spectra generated from the database.
- A correlation score is calculated for each match between the MS-MS scan and the theoretical MS-MS spectra.

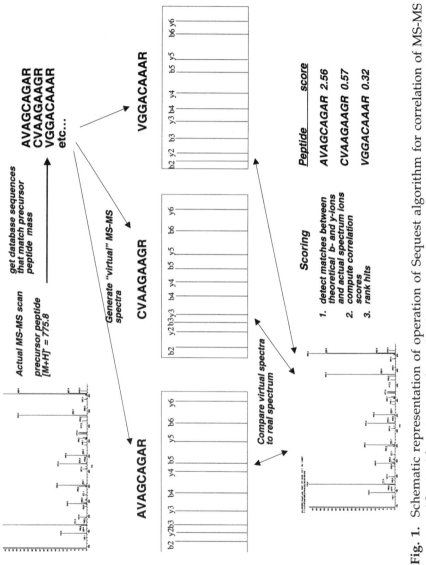

Fig. 1. Schematic representation of operation of Sequest algorithm for correlation of MS-MS

The best match or matches for each MS-MS scan analyzed is then reported. The results for the analyses of all the MS-MS scans in a datafile (e.g., an LC-MS-MS run) are presented in a web-browser-based window. A summary of the peptide sequences matched to MS-MS spectra for any particular protein is also displayed (**Fig. 2**). The quality of the matches of individual MS-MS scans to database entries can be evaluated on the basis of the correlation scores reported or by visual inspection of the actual MS-MS spectra overlaid with the predicted b- and/or y-ions from the "best match" peptide. This makes it relatively easy to distinguish reliable matches from unreliable ones. For example, an MS-MS spectrum in which over half of the predicted b- and y-ions in a peptide match the major signals in the spectrum is often a correct match (**Fig. 3**). On the other hand, a spectrum in which most of the prominent fragment ions do not match the purported b- and y-ions for the putative peptide is usually an incorrect match (**Fig. 4**).

However, it is important to realize that Sequest does not make judgments about the quality of the matches assigned. The algorithm will identify the best peptide sequence match in the database to each MS-MS scan analyzed—even if the match is of very poor quality. Thus, the user must use some combination of knowledge and intuition to decide which matches to accept and which to reject. One aid to decision-making is a summary of database proteins matched to MS-MS scans, which is presented in the browser window, which lists the proteins in order of decreasing numbers of hits (i.e., MS-MS scan matches). A protein with several high-quality hits on different peptide sequences is likely to be correctly identified. On the other hand, a protein with one or two weak matches to MS-MS spectra may not be correctly identified. The most reliable protein identifications are those in which several different sequences within the identified protein provide high-quality matches to MS-MS spectra in the datafile.

There are a number of complications that can make Sequest analyses more time-consuming or less accurate and complete. First, many peptides bear covalent modifications, which modify the m/z values of the peptides actually analyzed. Thus, Sequest would use a mass that did not correspond to the unmodified peptide mass in the database. In this case, no correct match between the MS-MS scan of the modified peptide and the database sequence would be possible because of this

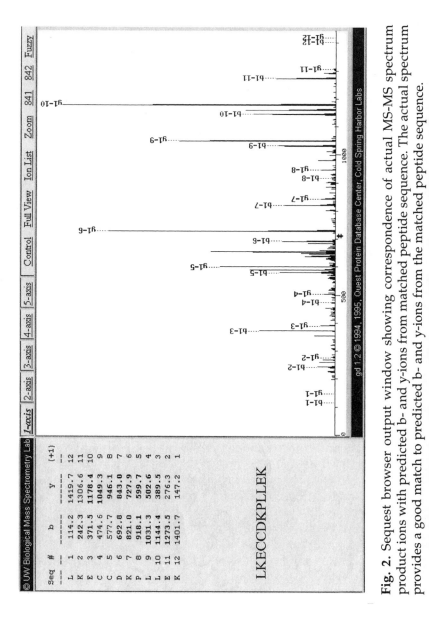

Fig. 2. Sequest browser output window showing correspondence of actual MS-MS spectrum product ions with predicted b- and y-ions from matched peptide sequence. The actual spectrum provides a good match to predicted b- and y-ions from the matched peptide sequence.

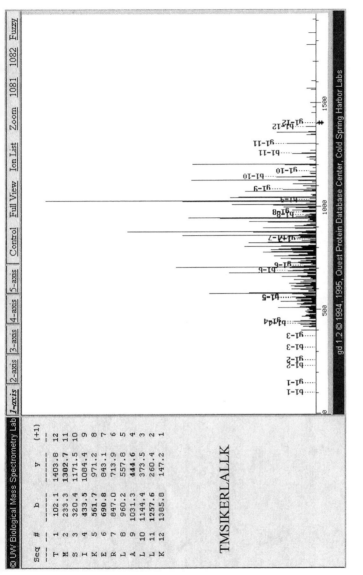

Fig. 3. Sequest browser output window showing correspondence of actual MS-MS spectrum productions with predicted b- and y-ions from matched peptide sequence. The actual spectrum provides a poor match to predicted b- and y-ions from the matched peptide sequence.

105

```
>gi|418694|pir||ABBOS serum albumin precursor [validated] - bovine [MASS=69270]
MKWVTFISLL LLFSSAYSRG VFRRDTHKSE IAHRFKDLGE EQFKGLVLIA FSQYLQQCPF DEHVKLVNEL TEFAKTCVAD
ESHAGCEKSL HTLFGDELCK VASLRETYGD MADCCEKQEP ERNECFLSHK DDSPDLPKLK PDPNTLCDEF KADEKKFWGK
YLYEIARRHP YFYAPELLYY ANKYNGVFQD CCQAEDKGAC LLPKIETMRE KVLASSARQR LRCASIQKFG ERALKAWSVA
RLSQKFPKAE FVEVTKLVTD LTKVHKECCH GDLLECADDR ADLAKYICDN QDTISSKLKE CCDKPLLEKS HCIAEVEKDA
IPENLPPLTA DFAEDKDVCK NYQEAKDAFL GSFLYEYSRR HPEYAVSVLL RLAKEYEATL EECCAKDDPH ACYSTVFDKL
KHLVDEPQNL IKQNCDQFEK LGEYGFQNAL IVRYTRKVPQ VSTPTLVEVS RSLGKVGTRC CTKPESERMP CTEDYLSLIL
NRLCVLHEKT PVSEKVTKCC TESLVNRRPC FSALTPDETY VPKAFDEKLF TFHADICTLP DTEKQIKKQT ALVELLKHKP
KATEEQLKTV MENFVAFVDK CCAADDKEAC FAVEGPKLVV STQTALA
```

Mass (average): 69270.4   Identifier: gi|418694   Database: C:/Xcalibur/database/bovine.fasta
Protein Coverage: 232/607 = 38.2% by amino acid count, 26178.1/69270.4 = 37.8% by mass

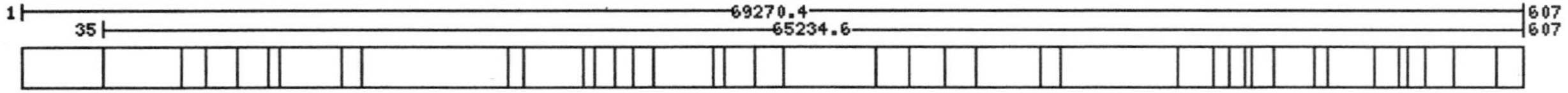

Fig. 4. Sequest browser output window depicting sequence coverage for matched protein based on correlation of MS-MS spectra to peptide sequences.

106

mass difference. To deal with this problem, Sequest allows the user to specify specific modifications to amino acids, such that the algorithm can search for both the modified and unmodified variants. This works reasonably well with anticipated modifications (e.g., phosphorylation of serine, threonine, or tyrosine). However, unanticipated modifications nevertheless are common and may be missed. Another problem in Sequest analyses is incorrect assignment of charge state (e.g., singly vs. doubly charged ions) to precursor ions for MS-MS spectra. If a singly charged ion is incorrectly designated as doubly charged, it will be compared to theoretical MS-MS spectra from database peptides of the wrong mass. The same problem would ensue from incorrect designation of a doubly charged ion as singly charged.

These concerns are worth noting, but they should not distract us from the tremendous value of such a tool. The analysis of a datafile containing approx 2000 MS-MS scans with Sequest can be accomplished in less than an hour, depending on the database and computing platform used. The quality of protein matches provided by Sequest can be assessed sometimes within minutes and often within an hour or two of data review. This contrasts with the hundreds to thousands of hours it would take to perform manually *de novo* interpretation and BLAST search of the putative sequences. Thus Sequest and similar programs offer the user the capability to rapidly evaluate large amounts of LC-MS-MS data to identify proteins. When combined with automated LC-MS-MS instrument control (e.g., data-dependent scanning) and automated sample-preparation methods, Sequest and similar tools permit the automated, high-throughput identification of proteins.

9.3. Other Algorithms and Software Tools for Identifying Proteins from ESI Tandem MS Data

The general approach of comparing MS-MS spectral data with theoretical MS-MS spectra from peptide sequences is used in other algorithms and software tools. The MS-Tag program (http://prospector.ucsf.edu) was originally developed for analysis of PSD spectra obtained in MALDI-TOF analyses of peptides (*see* Chapter 6), but has been modified to accommodate MS-MS data from different types of instruments. The user can enter a list of m/z values from the MS-MS spectrum to be analyzed, the m/z value and charge state of the precursor ion, information about the type of enzyme used for proteolytic digestion, and information on the instrument used to obtain the MS-MS data. The algorithm prefilters the database for peptides that match the precursor m/z of the MS-MS spectrum being analyzed. The output provides a tabular list of matching peptides and fragments that matched the ions recorded in the actual MS-MS spectrum. MS-Tag is particularly well-suited to the analysis of MALDI-TOF PSD spectra, which contain immonium ions (low m/z fragments indicating the presence of individual amino acids).

The Mascot program (http://www.matrixscience.com/) uses the probability based MOWSE algorithm (*see* Chapter 7), precursor m/z information, and MS-MS fragment ion data to identify proteins from databases. Mascot is actually a cluster of programs that can be used for peptide mass fingerprinting (*see* Chapter 7) as well as analysis of MS-MS data. Automated input of multiple MS-MS spectra from LC-MS-MS datafiles can be achieved with the aid of conversion programs available on the Mascot website. A similar utility, PepFrag is available at http://prowl.rockefeller.edu/PROWL/pepfragch.html.

Suggested Reading

Clauser, K. R., Baker, P., and Burlingame, A. L. (1999) Role of accurate mass measurement (+/- 10 ppm) in protein identification strategies employing MS or MS/MS and database searching. *Anal. Chem.* **71,** 2871–2882.

Yates, J. R., Eng, J. K., and McCormack, A. L. (1995) Mining genomes: correlating tandem mass spectra of modified and unmodified peptides to sequences in nucleotide databases. *Anal. Chem.* **67,** 3202–3210.

Yates, J. R., Eng, J. K., McCormack, A. L., and Schieltz, D. (1995) Method to correlate tandem mass spectra of modified peptides to amino acid sequences in the protein database. *Anal. Chem.* **67,** 1426–1436.

10 SALSA: An Algorithm for Mining Specific Features of Tandem MS Data

10.1. Beyond Protein Identification

When using Sequest and similar tools described in previous chapters, we typically have peptide MS-MS data and we ask, "What proteins do these peptides come from?" Sequest and similar programs are well-suited to the task of protein identification from peptide MS-MS data. However, the proposition becomes a bit different if we want to do something other than simply identify what proteins are present in a sample. Consider the following scenarios:

- We know that our sample contains many proteins, but we only wish to identify those that bear some specific modification. This could be a posttranslational modification, such as phosphorylation, or a modification by a drug or other chemical.
- We want to identify peptides in a mixture that all share some sequence identity, but may differ in other ways. This could be due to the presence of wild-type and mutant forms of a protein.
- We know or suspect that our sample contains a particular protein, but we also suspect that it may be present in multiple modified forms and we wish to detect all of them.

As we will discuss in the following chapters, these scenarios are commonly encountered in real-life proteomic analyses. In each case, we do not want simply to identify everything in the mixture; we are

From: *Introduction to Proteomics: Tools for the New Biology*
By: D. C. Liebler © Humana Press, Inc., Totowa, NJ

instead asking for information on specific components of the sample. What we have are large numbers of MS-MS spectra obtained from the many different peptides in the sample. What we want to do is identify those MS-MS spectra that display the specific features of interest. In the first scenario, we are looking for spectra that indicate the presence of some specific functional group, such as a phosphorylated amino acid. In the second and third scenarios, we are looking for the MS-MS spectra that display b- or y-ion series that indicate a particular amino acid sequence motif, even if that motif may be present in several different peptides. To address these three scenarios, an algorithm called SALSA (Scoring ALgorithm for Spectral Analysis) can be employed.

10.2. The SALSA Algorithm

SALSA detects specific features in MS-MS spectra and scores the spectra based on how many of the features are displayed and their intensities in the spectrum. SALSA can detect four different types of features in MS-MS spectra (**Fig. 1**). The first is a *product ion* at a specific m/z value. An example is the loss of a chemical modification as a charged fragment that then appears in the MS-MS spectrum at a particular m/z value, regardless of the m/z of the peptide from which it was lost. The second is a *neutral loss*, in which a neutral fragment is lost from the precursor ion. The product ion has the same charge state as the precursor (e.g., a doubly charged ion will lose a neutral fragment to yield a doubly charged product ion). However, the difference between the mass of the precursor and the product ion detected will equal the mass of the lost neutral fragment. The third feature is a *charged loss*, in which a multiply charged precursor ion loses a charged fragment. An example of this is the loss of a singly charged fragment from a doubly charged precursor. Of course, the formation of singly charged b- and y-ions in MS-MS of doubly charged peptide ions is the most widely observed example of this. However, other variants of this process can be highly diagnostic for some chemical modifications. The fourth feature is an *ion pair*, which denotes any two signals separated by a specified m/z value anywhere in the MS-MS spectrum. The appearance of an ion pair can indicate the presence of a specific component in a peptide sequence. For example, the y-ion series in a cysteine-containing peptide would contain a pair of product ion signals separated by 103 m/z units due to the residue mass of cysteine.

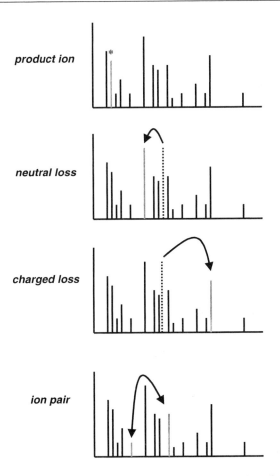

product ion

neutral loss

charged loss

ion pair

Fig. 1. Spectral characteristics detected by the SALSA algorithm.

These features or combinations of these features the MS-MS spectrum can be indicators of specific structural features in the precursor peptide. In principle, one could inspect individual MS-MS spectra from some analysis to determine whether specific features are present. However, the frequent need to examine hundreds or thousands of MS-MS spectra from a single LC-MS run makes this impractical, to say the least. We face the same problem we faced in trying to identify proteins from LC tandem MS analyses of complex peptide mixtures: there are too many spectra to evaluate by hand. Thus an algorithm such as SALSA serves the need to perform rapid computer-assisted screening of many MS-MS spectra rapidly.

Of course, merely detecting spectral features in not enough. An algorithm to identify the handful of MS-MS spectra that contain specific features in a datafile with hundreds of thousands of MS-MS scans must be able to rank the best hits. SALSA scores MS-MS scans based on the intensities of the ions that define the specified features. Thus, an MS-MS scan with an intense product ion arising from a specified neutral loss (e.g., loss of phosphoric acid from phosphoserine) would get a high score. In contrast, a relatively low-abundance product ion corresponding to the same neutral loss in another MS-MS scan would give that scan a low score.

An important feature of SALSA is its flexibility. The user can specify detection and scoring of those characteristics most closely associated with the peptide structural features of interest. As we shall see in subsequent chapters, neutral losses are highly indicative of certain posttranslational modifications (e.g., phosphorylation), whereas ion pairs are characteristic of others (some stable amino acid modifications), and still others are most clearly indicated by product ions (some drug or chemical modifications).

Another aspect of flexibility in SALSA scoring is the ability of the user to set a hierarchy of importance for different characteristics. Thus, some spectral features can be designated as primary characteristics and others as secondary. Primary characteristics are scored whenever they are detected. Secondary features are linked to some primary feature and are only scored when the linked primary feature is detected. For example, some chemical moieties (e.g., carbohydrates) that can modify peptides undergo a neutral loss of water, which in some cases can be diagnostic for a specific feature. However, a SALSA search for MS-MS scans that display a neutral loss of 18 mass units from the precursor is likely to turn up many hits. This is simply because it is highly likely that many peptide ions could fragment this way (such as those containing serine or threonine residues), even if they do not contain the structural feature of interest. However, one can make scoring of the neutral loss of water (18 amu) secondary to detection of some primary characteristic that is more unusual, such as some product ion or other, more unique neutral loss. Then the 18 amu loss is only scored in scans that contain the other characteristic as well and the two characteristics both contribute to the score for that scan. The use of multiple scoring criteria in a primary-secondary scoring hierarchy increases the ability of SALSA to detect selectively MS-MS scans derives from specific peptides and their derivatives.

10.3. Amino Acid Sequence-Motif Searching with SALSA

One of the key MS-MS features detected by SALSA is the appearance of an ion pair somewhere in the spectrum that is separated by some specified distance on the m/z axis. One of the most common sources of ion pairs in MS-MS spectra are b- and y- series ions. For example, the y-ion series for the AVAGCAGAR peptide discussed in Chapter 8 contains a pair of ions at m/z 477 and m/z 374, which are the y_5 and y_4 ions. These two ions are separated by a distance of 103 units on the m/z axis, which is indicative of the presence of a cysteine residue. Likewise, the y_4 and y_3 ions are separated by a gap of 71 m/z units, which corresponds to a valine residue. If we use ion pair searching to detect MS-MS scans with an ion pair separated by 103 units, SALSA can detect the MS-MS scan from AVAGCAGAR. However, it will likely also detect the MS-MS scans from just about every other cysteine-containing peptide in the sample. Of course, we could focus on the gap between y_5 and y_3, which corresponds to the cysteine and the alanine residues together and is 174 m/z units in length. This would perhaps be somewhat more selective and would pick out MS-MS scans of peptides containing a CV or VC dipeptide. However, it quickly would become evident that a single ion pair can never be a highly selective means of differentiating any one MS-MS scan from all the rest.

Indeed, the best approach to find the MS-MS spectrum of a particular peptide would be to detect not just a pair of ions but a *series* of ions. For example, if one could search through all the MS-MS spectra in a datafile for those that displayed a series of ions that matched some subset of a particular b- or y-ion series, the chances to detecting the MS-MS spectrum of the corresponding peptide would be greatly enhanced. Indeed, SALSA can be used to detect *ion series* in MS-MS spectra.

For a closer look at ion-series scoring, we again consider our familiar example peptide AVAGCAGAR. Let's assume that we have a datafile with several hundred MS-MS scans, one of which is for the doubly charged ion of AVAGCAGAR. How will we use ion-series searching to find it? We can begin by recalling that in most peptide MS-MS spectra, the most intense ions are those due to cleavages near the middle of the peptide. This means that we will want to search an ion series focused on the middle part of the peptide. We can start with the tripeptide sequence GCA, which corresponds to four ions (**Fig. 2**). Using the highest mass ion as a reference, the next ion in the series is 57 units lower (the glycine residue mass). The third is 103 units lower than the second (the cysteine residue mass) and the fourth is another 71 units lower than the third (the alanine residue mass). An ion series of this type would correspond to a y-ion series for a peptide containing a GCA motif. As depicted in **Fig. 2**, the specified ion series becomes a virtual "ruler" with tick-marks that can be matched to each MS-MS spectrum in a datafile. In **Fig. 2A**, the "GCA" ruler matches signals in the MS-MS spectrum of AVAGCAGAR. It is important to emphasize at this point that the ions in the series must be linked together, rather than be detected as separate pairs. A peptide that contains a glycine, cysteine, and alanine, but not in this same sequence will not match. This is illustrated in **Fig. 2B**, in which the MS-MS spectrum of the peptide AVACAGGAR does not match the "GCA" ruler as well, even though the peptide has the same amino acid composition. The peptide contains a rearranged sequence with a "CAG" motif instead of a "GCA" motif in the middle. This displaces two of the ions in the y_3-y_4-y_5-y_6 series (i.e., y_4 and y_5) such that they do not match the ruler. Note that the y_3 and y_6 ions do match, as they define the ends of the series and the amino acid composition of the rearranged motif and the original motif are the same.

The only problem with doing an ion-series search for a short-sequence motif is that other peptides containing the GCA motif may be detected as well. However, a search of the VAGCAGA motif (an eight-ion series) is much more likely to identify selectively the MS-MS scan for the AVAGCAGAR peptide.

An important convention in SALSA is that the ions in a series are entered from the highest m/z to the lowest. Thus, a search with the VAGCAGA motif starts with a gap of 99 units between the first two

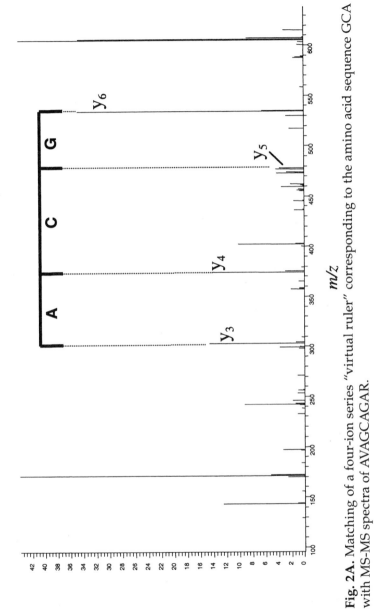

A

AVAGCAGAR

Fig. 2A. Matching of a four-ion series "virtual ruler" corresponding to the amino acid sequence GCA with MS-MS spectra of AVAGCAGAR.

115

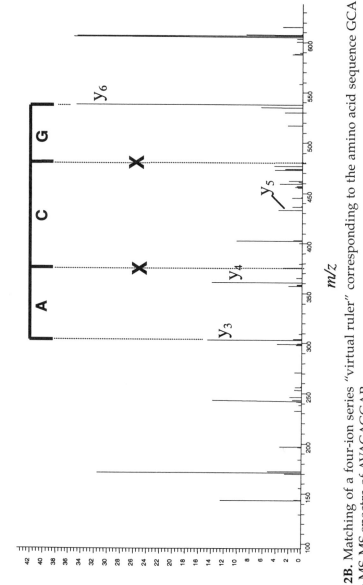

Fig. 2B. Matching of a four-ion series "virtual ruler" corresponding to the amino acid sequence GCA with MS-MS spectra of AVACAGGAR.

ions (valine), followed by a gap of 71 units to the next (alanine), then a gap of 57 units to the next (glycine) and so forth. This series of ions corresponds to the y-ion series for the AVAGCAGAR peptide (**Fig. 3**). The highest mass ion would correspond to the y-ion [VAGCAGAR + H]$^+$ at m/z 703.82 (note that this ion is not seen in the spectrum in **Fig. 3**). The next ion in the series would correspond to [AGCAGAR + H]$^+$ at m/z 604.69, the next to [GCAGAR + H]$^+$ at m/z 533.61, and so forth. In MS-MS spectra of tryptic peptides, the y-ion series is often more intense than the b-ion series (although there are frequent exceptions to this rule of thumb). Of course, one could search the ion series corresponding to AGACGAV, which would match the b-ion series for the AVAGCAGAR peptide.

SALSA scores MS-MS spectra for ion series based on: 1) the number of ions in the MS-MS spectrum that match the series, and 2) the intensities of the ions that are matched. MS-MS spectra that have intense signals that match most or all of the ions in the series will get the highest scores. On the other hand, those MS-MS spectra that matches only a few of the ions in the series or those in which the matched ions are of low intensity will get low scores. The user may control the stringency of the match by specifying a minimum number of ions that must be found in the MS-MS spectrum for a match.

10.4. Applications of Ion-Series Detection with SALSA

The utility of ion-series detection can be illustrated with two examples. In the first, we are interested in detecting two variant forms of a protein. One is a wild-type sequence, whereas the other has a single amino acid substitution. Tryptic digestion of the wild-type protein yields a peptide AVAGCAGAR, whereas the mutant yields a peptide AVAGCAVAR. Let's assume we have done an LC-tandem MS analysis of a tryptic digest containing these two peptides and we wish to find the MS-MS scans corresponding to both. The relatively subtle change in sequence (substitution of valine for glycine at position 7) nevertheless changes the y-ion series. Specifically, the y-ions y_3–y_7 are displaced by the mass difference between glycine and valine, such that these y ions appear at higher m/z in the spectrum of AVAGCAVAR (**Fig. 4A** vs **4B**). The "ruler" defined by the sequence motif AGCA matches the series in both the top and bottom spectra, even though the

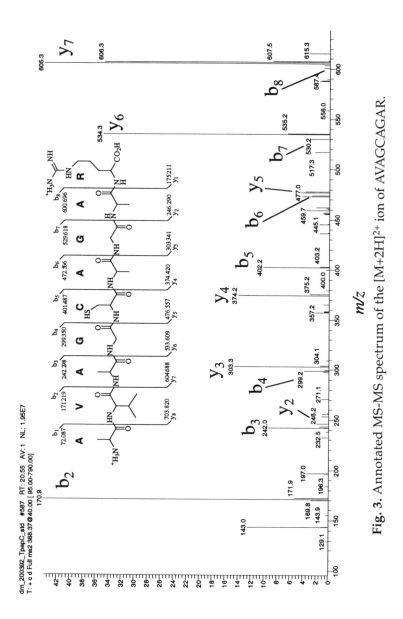

Fig. 3. Annotated MS-MS spectrum of the [M+2H]²⁺ ion of AVAGCAGAR.

ions detected appear at different absolute m/z values. Nevertheless, the *relative* positions of the ions in the series are the same in both spectra. Thus, a SALSA search for AGCA should detect both peptides.

Ion-series searching is tolerant of small variations. If we searched the MS-MS spectra of AVAGCAGAR and AVAGCAVAR instead with the series AGCAG, we would also detect both peptides (**Fig. 4**). However, the match to the MS-MS spectrum for AVAGCAGAR would be better than the match for the MS-MS spectrum for AVAGCAVAR, because the AGCAG "ruler" would detect the y_2–y_7 ions for AVAGCAGAR, but only the y_3–y_7 ions for AVAGCAVAR (compare **Fig. 4A** and **4B**). Despite this small difference, MS-MS scans for both peptides would be detected with higher scores than MS-MS scans for other peptides that lack the specified sequence motif entirely.

A second example of the utility of ion-series searching with SALSA is the detection of products from incomplete proteolytic digestion. The failure of proteolytic enzymes to cleave with perfect efficiency is a fact of life in proteomics. If our AVAGCAGAR peptide was part of a larger sequence . . . FPGKYKAVAGCAGARTGKH . . ., we might expect that incomplete digestion also would yield YKAVAGCAGAR and AVAGCAGARTGK. The y-ion series (from y_1–y_8) for YKAVAGCAGAR would be identical to that for AVAGCAGAR, although the former would also include y_9 and y_{10} ions. A search for ion series corresponding to VAGCAGA would pick up MS-MS scans for both peptides. What is particularly useful about SALSA is that the same search would also pick up the MS-MS scan for the AVAGCAGARTGK peptide. Because this peptide contains a C-terminal extension (relative to AVAGCAGAR), its y-ions fall at different m/z values in the MS-MS spectrum. However, the spacing of the gaps in the series defined by the search sequence VAGCAGA remains the same, albeit shifted along the m/z axis.

This scenario again underscores the power of ion-series searching with the SALSA algorithm. The application of a pattern-recognition algorithm to the evaluation of MS-MS data allows the selective detection of MS-MS scans corresponding to essentially any peptide sequence or modified peptide and variants thereof. Of course, the MS-MS scans thus detected provide the most unambiguous proof that those peptides were present in the mixture analyzed and, in turn, in the protein samples from which they came.

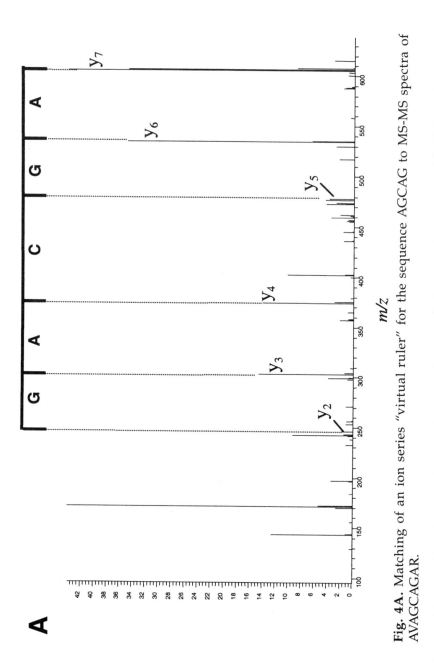

Fig. 4A. Matching of an ion series "virtual ruler" for the sequence AGCAG to MS-MS spectra of AVAGCAGAR.

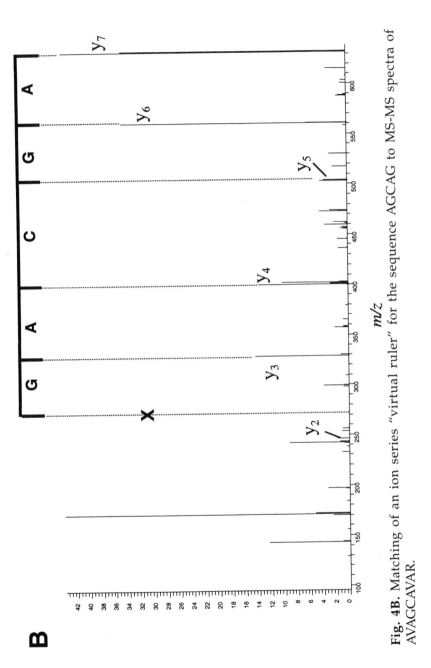

Fig. 4B. Matching of an ion series "virtual ruler" for the sequence AGCAG to MS-MS spectra of AVAGCAVAR.

121

Suggested Reading

Hansen, B. T., Jones, J. A., Mason, D. E., and Liebler, D. C. (2001) SALSA: a pattern recognition algorithm to detect electrophile-adducted peptides by automated evaluation of CID spectra in LC-MS-MS analyses. *Anal. Chem.* **73,** 1676–1683.

Liebler, D. C., Hansen, B. T., Davey, S. W., Tiscareno, L., and Mason, D. E. (2001) Peptide sequence motif analysis of tandem ms data with the SALSA algorithm. *Anal. Chem.*, in press.

III Applications of Proteomics

11 Mining Proteomes

11.1. One Genome, Many Proteomes

The purpose of proteome mining is to identify as many of the components of the proteome as possible. In our previous discussions, we have considered "the proteome" as if it were a complete protein complement of all of the organism's genes. However, this "master" proteome is something of an abstraction. No cell in any organism contains all proteins encoded by its genes all together at one time. Even in yeast, about a third of the yeast genome is not expressed at any given time.

In higher organisms, different genes and proteins are expressed in different tissues and at different stages of development. For example, retinal pigment epithelium in the eye and aortic smooth muscle certainly express many proteins in common, particularly those associated with essential cellular functions. However, expression of contractile proteins is characteristic of the muscle, whereas expression of photoreceptors is characteristic of the retinal pigment epithelium. In stimulated muscle or light-exposed retinal pigment epithelium, more subtle changes occur, including changes in protein expression or posttranslational modification. Thus, different cells express different proteomes and the same cell may express different proteomes in different states.

In addition to the many proteomes of different cells in an organism, there are other interesting, unique proteomes in organisms. Extracellular fluids contain many secreted proteins. Blood plasma, CSF, saliva, urine, and sweat all contain proteomes that change in response to

From: *Introduction to Proteomics: Tools for the New Biology*
By: D. C. Liebler © Humana Press, Inc., Totowa, NJ

the state of an organism. What is interesting about these proteomes is that changes in their protein composition may be associated with disease processes in the organism and thus have potential utility as diagnostic markers. The key point is that any proteome is defined by the state of the organism, tissue, or cell that produces it. Because these states are constantly changing, so are the proteomes.

11.2. Selecting Proteomes for Analysis

If we accept the proposition that different cells and tissues contain different proteomes, then we must consider cell and tissue sampling as the first consideration in selective proteome analysis. To characterize a proteome, we want to obtain a cell or tissue sample that is as homogeneous and representative of that cell or tissue type as possible. In some cases, as with cultured cells, this may be relatively straightforward. If one wishes to analyze a complex tissue such as the mammalian kidney, there are many cell types in close juxtaposition to each other. There are techniques for dissociating and fractionating cells from tissues and they may be applied to such situations. However, changes in the biochemistry of the target cells during workup may significantly perturb the system. One recently introduced technique for selectively sampling certain cells within a tissue is *laser-capture microdissection*, which couples microscopy to tissue harvesting and allows the user to extract selectively certain cells from frozen sections of tissue. This permits the analyst to select the population of cells to be subjected to further analysis. Application of laser-capture microdissection to the analysis of tumors and adjacent normal tissues has facilitated recent studies of gene-expression changes in cancer. The problem with capturing small amounts of tissue or cells for analysis is that there is less total protein to work with. Accordingly, it is far more difficult to detect less abundantly expressed proteins in smaller tissue samples.

Another important point in tissue or cell sampling is that isolation procedures often induce cellular stresses and the proteome may change in response to these stresses. The increased formation of reactive oxygen species (ROS) during cell sampling and DNA extraction is a well-known artifact that complicates the analysis of oxidative damage in vivo. Because ROS can also oxidize proteins and activate adaptive responses, the potential for artifactual alterations in the proteome is significant, particularly for stress-associated gene products. A second major concern during cell homogenization and fractionation is the activation of endogenous proteases, which may cleave many proteins to fragments. Although proteomic analysis of the fragments may still yield useful information, attempts to link the acquired data to fractions based on molecular weight may be confusing. Finally, the manner in which a tissue sample is prepared and stored can greatly affect the success of proteomic analysis. Fixed tissue samples are generally inappropriate for proteomic analysis because tissue treatment with formaldehyde or some similar fixative cross-links proteins and prevents both the digestion and the recovery of any peptide fragments. In contrast, frozen sections can be very amenable to protein analysis.

Despite these concerns regarding the perils of fractionation, there is one overriding advantage to fractionating proteomes for analysis: it simplifies them. Remember that our ability to detect multiple protein species in a sample depends on our ability to resolve many peptides from the sample and obtain MS data on as many of them as possible. Selection of a subcellular fraction (e.g., the mitochondria) for analysis reduces the task from analysis of perhaps 25,000 proteins in a human cell sample to analysis of about 1000–2000. With current technology, we have a better chance of identifying less abundant proteins when they are present in a mixture of 1000 proteins than when they are in a mixture of 15,000 proteins. Consequently, the best current approach to proteome analysis in a cell or tissue sample may be to fractionate the sample first either on the basis of subcellular fractions. For simpler proteomes (e.g., CSF) such a prefractionation may be unnecessary.

11.3. Mining Approach #1: 2D-SDS-PAGE and MALDI-TOF MS

In this approach we combine a powerful protein separation method (2D-SDS-PAGE) with a convenient, high-throughput MS analytical method (MALDI-TOF MS). The overall approach is sketched out in **Fig. 1**. Proteins are first extracted from the sample and then separated by 2D-SDS-PAGE (*see* Chapter 4). The protein spots can then be visualized by staining. Manual inspection of the spots can be bewildering, so it is convenient to use an imaging system to record an image of the stained gel to provide a record of the protein distribution in the

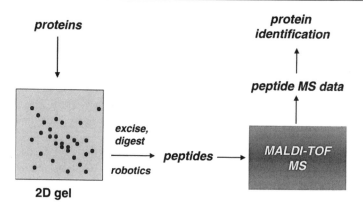

Fig. 1. Schematic representation of proteome mining by 2D-SDS-PAGE and MALDI-TOF MS.

sample. These images can be analyzed, compared, and archived with several available software packages. Because the purpose of mining is to identify as many system components as possible, many or all of the spots can be selected and cut from the gel. In-gel digestion is used to cleave the proteins to peptides, which then are analyzed by MALDI-TOF MS (*see* Chapters 6 and 7). The MS data then are analyzed with the aid of a peptide mass fingerprinting algorithm and software (*see* Chapter 7), which identifies the proteins present.

As noted earlier, the advantages of this approach are the separation power of the 2D gel and the throughput, sensitivity, and convenience of MALDI-TOF MS for protein identification. Typical analyses of proteomes by this approach yield identification of about 50–75% of the proteins in the selected spots, depending on several things.

Higher identification yields are typical of organisms with smaller proteomes (e.g., bacteria or yeast) compared to higher organisms. This is because these organisms have fewer genes overall and fewer near-identical members (paralogs) within distinct gene families (*see* Chapter 2). In contrast, higher organisms such as *D. melanogaster* and *C. elegans* have greater numbers of protein paralogs, which may yield a number of identical peptides in addition to any that are different. This reduces the confidence of a match made on the basis of one or two unique peptides.

Another problem with peptide mass fingerprinting approaches to protein identification is the uncertainty of annotation of published genome sequences. The coding sequences of the many genes in a sequenced genome are initially assigned by algorithms that help define the beginning and end of each gene-coding sequence. The algorithms that make these assignments have significant error rates, which may approach 30% or more. Thus, the bulk of the coding sequence may be correct, but the uncertainty will introduce error into mass fingerprinting involving the N- and C-terminal peptides. This problem will gradually recede as the annotation of genome sequences progresses and the mass fingerprinting algorithms can be used with completed protein-sequence databases. A related problem is that genome sequences do not necessarily predict splice variants, which may be significant forms of some proteins. Again, some peptides may be identical between two forms of a protein, but variant peptides will cause uncertainty in protein assignment by the peptide mass fingerprinting algorithms.

Another concern regarding the use of 2D gels as the front end for this approach is that, despite their resolving power, 2D gels do not completely resolve all proteins into single spots. Indeed, many spots contain 2–5 proteins, depending on the nature of the sample and the location of the spots on the gel. Digestion of these multiprotein spots yields mixtures of peptides from two or more proteins and this again introduces uncertainty in the assignment of corresponding proteins by mass fingerprinting software tools. Although the newer algorithms can assign multiple protein components to MALDI-TOF spectra of peptide mixtures, the error in assignment can increase significantly with increasing complexity of the mixture.

A final concern with this approach to proteome mining is that 2D-SDS-PAGE, even with the most sensitive stains available, exhibits a limited dynamic range for protein detection. Cellular expression levels of different proteins can differ by as much as a million-fold. However, the dynamic range for protein staining in 2D gels is about a hundred- to a thousand-fold at best. Thus, 2D gels typically detect only the most abundantly expressed proteins. Recent careful analyses of the yeast proteome by this approach indicated that only about 1500 of 4000+ expressed proteins could be detected and that these proteins were the products of the most highly expressed genes. Thus, the

2D-SDS-PAGE and MALDI-TOF approach to proteome mining misses a lot, including many proteins of biological significance.

11.4. Mining Approach #2: Multidimensional Peptide Chromatography and LC-Tandem MS Analysis

A second approach to proteome mining blends multidimensional peptide separations with the power of peptide sequence identification by tandem MS. The approach is sketched out in **Fig. 2**. In this approach, one begins by digesting the proteins in the mixture to peptides (*see* Chapter 5). The peptides are resolved (at least partially) by chromatography and then electrospray tandem MS is used to obtain MS-MS spectra of the peptides (*see* Chapters 8 and 9). These spectra are then mapped to protein sequences from databases with the aid of Sequest or similar search tools (*see* Chapter 9).

There are several variants of this basic approach, but its two distinguishing characteristics are: 1) the analysis primarily involves working with peptides rather than with proteins; and 2) protein identification is based on the MS-MS fragmentation spectra, rather than on peptide mass fingerprinting. In the most basic version of this approach, no attempt is made to first separate the proteins in the mixture from each other. However, the peptides generated by digestion of the protein mixture may be resolved by different LC steps prior to MS.

The basic idea with this approach is to acquire MS-MS spectra for as many of the peptides in the mixture as possible. Recall that tandem MS instruments used for proteomic analyses typically use data-dependent control of the instrument to select peptide ions for MS-MS and record the data. To maximize the number of different peptides analyzed, it helps to "spread out" the peptide mixture as much as possible. To do this, let's consider the simplest LC-MS approach to peptide analysis and then several variations:

1. RP LC-MS only. In this approach, the peptide mixture is analyzed by RP LC-MS with elution by a water/acetonitrile gradient. Resolution of the peptides in the mixture is achieved by the RP LC gradient separation. This is the simplest system. It works well unless the peptide mixture is complex enough that there are more than perhaps five different peptides eluting from the column at

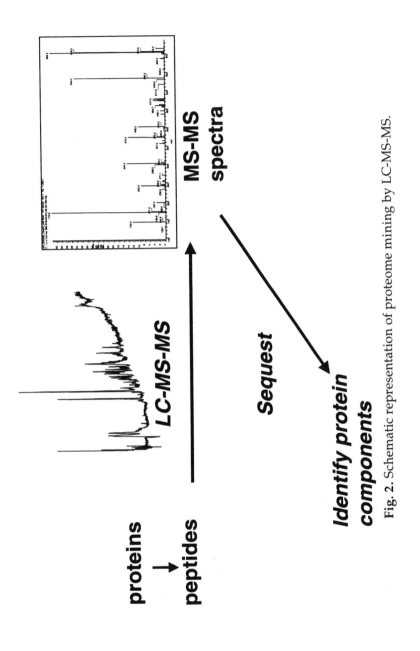

proteins → peptides

LC-MS-MS

MS-MS spectra

Sequest

Identify protein components

Fig. 2. Schematic representation of proteome mining by LC-MS-MS.

any one time. When the mixture is more complex than that, the instrument simply cannot keep up with all the different peptides coming from the column and some pass by unrecorded. In that case, the instrument is most likely to obtain MS-MS spectra on approximately five of the most abundant peptide ions eluting in that time interval.

2. RP LC-MS with stop flow control. This approach is identical to that described earlier except that the MS instrument can sense when a "crowd" of peptides elutes from the column. In order to avoid missing some of the peptides, the system slows down the pump flow. This slows the elution of the "crowd" of peptide ions to give the MS more time to record MS-MS data on all the peptide ions. Specifically, when the total ion current exceeds some threshold value, the MS exerts feedback control on the LC pump to slow or stop flow. If a complex mixture of two dozen different peptides were eluting at that moment, the instrument would have time to obtain systematically MS-MS spectra on all of the peptides, rather than on the top five or six. This strategy, often called "peak parking," can be remarkably effective for increasing the number of peptide components characterized in a mixture. Setting up the feedback control system requires some instrument programming skill. Disadvantages of the approach stem from the many stops and starts caused by the stop-flow approach. The chromatography runs can be very long and can generate huge datafiles that can make even computer-assisted data analysis quite challenging. In addition, diffusion (band spreading) of the analytes on the column during the long runs gradually results in diminished chromatographic resolution.

3. Tandem LC-tandem MS (*see* Chapter 4, **Fig. 7**). This chromatographic approach was described in Chapter 4 and entails placing a strong cation exchange column in line immediately ahead of the RP column. The entire sample is then loaded onto the strong cation-exchange column, to which most of the peptides bind. A salt gradient step is used to elute the most loosely bound peptides, which then are resolved by an RP gradient. This cycle of salt step elution followed by RP is repeated 15–20 times. The net effect is a tremendous "spreading" of the peptide mixture by the two-phase chromatography system and a concomitant increase in

the number of peptides identified. As with the "peak parking" approach described earlier, the run times may be very long (6–18 h!) and the datafiles very large. Indeed, Yates and colleagues, who introduced this approach, have developed a special version of Sequest to use a computer cluster to analyze the data. A simpler variant of this approach described by Patterson and colleagues is to use a binary ion-exchange approach in which peptides that do not stick to the ion-exchange column are analyzed by RP LC-MS. Then a single salt pulse is used to elute the remaining peptides for a second RP LC-MS run. This produces a significant enhancement of detection for peptides without generating such large datafiles as in the multistep ion-exchange/RP cycles. Another variant of this approach is to use a stand-alone strong cation exchange column with a salt gradient to separate the peptides into groups. The collected salt gradient fractions are then analyzed sequentially by the simple RP LC-MS system described earlier in option 1.

4. There are a few other "tricks" that can be used to improve the performance of any of the three approaches described previously. First, one may realize that only peptides of between about 5 and 20 amino acids in length will generate useful MS-MS information for database-search algorithms. Thus, use of a size-exclusion chromatography step prior to LC-MS can limit the sample to only those peptides most likely to yield identifications. Another interesting idea manipulates the data-dependent instrument control system. It is possible to enter an "exclusion list," which is a list of ions the instrument will ignore (i.e., not subject to MS-MS analysis) during the run. Thus, one can run a sample once and the system will acquire MS-MS data for many, but not all of the peptides. At the end of the run, the list of ions just analyzed is then entered as the exclusion list and the sample is re-analyzed. The instrument now records data only for peptide ions that were not analyzed during the first run. This increases the total number of peptide ions for which MS-MS spectra are recorded during the two runs combined.

The LC-tandem MS approaches to proteome mining described previously all begin with a crude protein mixture that is digested to peptides and then analyzed. An attractive feature of this approach is the avoidance of difficult protein-separation techniques, such as those involving 2D gels. However, starting with a large collection of peptides from an unfractionated protein mixture does place a great burden on the peptide chromatography steps to "spread out" the mixture prior to MS analysis. One could lessen the burden on the downstream separations somewhat by adding a simple protein-fractionation step at the beginning of the sample workup. There are several different simple fraction steps one might employ to do this. Ion-exchange chromatography of the proteins in the mixture can be used to separate the proteins into anywhere from 5–20 fractions. Another similar approach is the use of solution-phase preparative IEF. Commercially available apparatus yield 12–20 fractions. A third possibility is the use of preparative 1D-SDS-PAGE. In each case, the separation can accommodate milligram to gram quantities of proteins. A high capacity for this step is important, because it increases the likelihood of detecting less abundantly expressed proteins in the final LC-MS analyses.

11.5. Which Approach is Best?

Both general approaches to proteome mining discussed earlier have distinct advantages. The use of 2D gels and MALDI-TOF MS offers high throughput and takes maximum advantage of powerful protein-separation methodology. The use of multidimensional LC-tandem MS analyses of peptides generates the most reliable protein identification because it is based on MS-MS spectra, which directly indicate peptide sequences. Both approaches present problems as well. Two-dimensional gels are difficult to reproduce and the 2D gel and MALDI-TOF MS approach is biased toward the detection of high-abundance proteins. On the other hand, the use of multidimensional LC separations with tandem MS is technically challenging and still rapidly evolving. Indeed, one's choice of approach may be dictated by the resources available. In either case, a great deal of progress can be made in proteome mining projects with either approach. In the best circumstances, both approaches can be used to provide complimentary information. Two-dimensional gels and MALDI-TOF MS are well-suited to somewhat simpler samples where the goal is to characterize major system components. It is also worth noting that changes in spot intensities in 2D SDS-PAGE offer an obvious means of comparing proteomes. This will be discussed further in the next chapter. However, for exhaustive mining of both high- and low-abundance proteins in complex mixtures, multidimensional LC combined with tandem MS clearly is the most effective approach. This conclusion is underscored by a careful comparison of the two approaches to mining the yeast proteome was recently published by Aebersold and colleagues. Because the approaches to proteome mining are evolving rapidly, it seems likely that technical refinements and novel combinations of protein separations will greatly enhance the effectiveness of the LC-MS approach by further "spreading out" complex peptide mixtures.

Suggested Reading

Davis, M. T., Beierle, J., Bures, E. T., McGinley, M. D., Mort, J., Robinson, J. H., Spahr, C. S., Yu, W., Luethy, R., and Patterson, S. D. (2001) Automated LC-LC-MS-MS platform using binary ion-exchange and gradient reversed-phase chromatography for improved proteomic analyses. *J. Chromatogr. B. Biomed. Sci. Appl.* **752,** 281–291.

Gygi, S. P., Corthals, G. L., Zhang, Y., Rochon, Y., and Aebersold, R. (2000) Evaluation of two-dimensional gel electrophoresis-based proteome analysis technology. *Proc. Natl. Acad. Sci. USA* **97,** 9390–9395.

Simone, N. L., Paweletz, C. P., Charboneau, L., Petricoin, E. F., and Liotta, L. A. (2000) Laser capture microdissection: beyond functional genomics to proteomics. *Mol. Diagn.* **5,** 301–307.

Washburn, M. P., Wolters, D., and Yates, J. R. (2001) Large-scale analysis of the yeast proteome by multidimensional protein identification technology. *Nat. Biotechnol.* **19,** 242–247

12 Protein Expression Profiling

12.1. The Changing Proteome

Much work in biochemistry and physiology already has shown us that biochemical pathways are constantly in flux. The use of DNA microarrays has demonstrated that gene-expression patterns in cells are also changing constantly. Indeed, one can use either old or new technologies to observe regular changes in the status of many enzymes during the daily life cycle of an organism or in the cycle of a cell. All this suggests that the proteomes of cells are constantly changing as well. In addition to these changes that are essential to life, other changes are induced by environmental stimuli, chemicals, drugs, and growth and disease processes. Many of these latter changes interest those trying to understand complicated pathologies (e.g., cancer) or trying to identify novel targets for therapeutic drugs. Perhaps the ultimate challenge of proteomics is to measure the status of all cellular proteins as they change with time. Unfortunately, the technology is not yet there. Nevertheless, the problem of comparing proteomes between two states of a cell or organism is relevant and important.

The most fundamental task in protein-expression profiling is to measure the expression of a set of proteins in two samples and then compare them. To do this, we simply need a method that detects and identifies the same proteins in the two samples and provides a basis for comparing their levels. This can be done in two different ways, as is outlined below. However, these methods may indicate

From: *Introduction to Proteomics: Tools for the New Biology*
By: D. C. Liebler © Humana Press, Inc., Totowa, NJ

only the level of the polypeptide gene product *per se*, but not how proteins are changed by modification. This requires not only use of the techniques outlined in this chapter, but also integration of the approaches outlined in subsequent chapters.

12.2. Comparative Proteomics with 2D Gels

Perhaps the most widely used approach to comparative proteomics is to subject two samples to 2D-SDS-PAGE and compare the spot patterns. Two-dimensional SDS-PAGE is particularly well-suited to comparative proteome analysis because it effectively resolves many proteins. With recent improvements in 2D gel technology (*see* Chapter 4), the task of running reproducible 2D gels has been made easier. Even before the introduction of MS-based protein identification, this approach provided a useful means of comparing proteomes. However, identification of the proteins was cumbersome and difficult. Application of peptide mass fingerprinting and LC-MS-MS analyses now makes it possible to identify essentially any protein one can detect by staining the gel. Thus, the critical task in comparative proteomics with 2D gels is identifying the features that differ between gels.

A great deal of work has been done to develop software tools to analyze the patterns of protein spots on 2D gels. In addition, extensive databases to archive this information have been developed. Among the most widely used programs for 2D gel-image analysis is Melanie™, which was developed at the Swiss Institute for Bioinformatics. Melanie™ works with images of stained 2D gels. These images can be acquired by use of a document scanner (to produce .gif or .tif files) or preferably by the use of a CCD camera. The program does several things. First, the gel is evaluated for "features," which simply refer to any significant deviation from the background. The features correspond to the protein spots on the gel (*see* **Fig. 1**). The features can be characterized by optical density (OD), by size, and by volume, which integrates OD over the spot area. These characteristics comprise the basis for comparing features within a gel and between multiple gels.

Of course, for protein-expression profiling, we want to compare the 2D gels from two different samples for differences in the occurrence or intensity of features. The problem with this is that it is very hard to run multiple 2D gels with exact reproducibility. There usually are

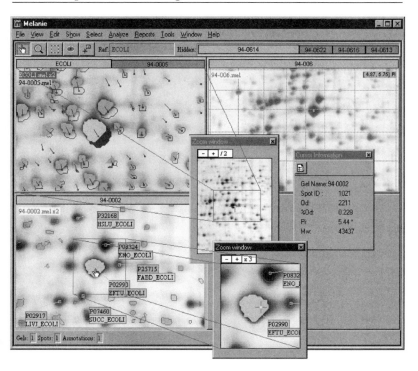

Fig. 1. Annotation of protein spot images on 2D gels with Melanie™ analysis software.

slight variations in the location of spots for specific proteins. This makes it hard to compare spots on two gels if their locations are slightly different. To accommodate these differences, the software allows the user to identify "landmarks," which are proteins that occur in both (or all) of the gels to be compared. These features then are "paired" by the software to create a series of pairs by which the gels can be aligned or "matched." The matching process involves alignment of the two gels so that the landmarks have the same relation to each other in 2D space. In other words, the gel images are lined up pixel-wise so that all the landmark features match. This process can entail some transformations or spatial "warping" of the images to compensate for local geometric distortions in the gel.

Once the gels are matched, then comparison of the features may be done. These comparisons examine the OD volume differences between features on the gels and provide a graphical output that assigns numbers to the observed differences (*see* **Fig. 2**). The software also enables statistical analyses of these data to facilitate interpretation of significant differences. It is this operation that allows the user to identify those features or spots that differ between two or more samples. Gels may be visually "stacked" to enable comparison of images. Alternatively, virtual gels can be synthesized from the images collected from multiple gels to provide a master archive of composite proteomes in different states of an organism.

Identification of the proteins in these spots of interest then involves excision of the spots, in-gel digestion, and MS analysis. In addition to detecting differences between features on multiple gels, the software also allows the user to annotate the features and to link them to database files containing MS data, gene sequences and functional genomics data.

The ability to compare two gels and then identify differently expressed spots is the essence of protein-expression profiling with 2D gels. However, the development of this approach by a number of groups has led to the development of 2D-SDS-PAGE databases, which archive large numbers of annotated images from 2D gel analyses. These databases are an increasingly powerful resource for the comparison of data generated in different laboratories. A powerful feature of these databases and software programs such as Melanie is the ability to compare large numbers of gels to a single gel or to groups of gels and compile statistical summaries of patterns in protein spot variation.

Another unique software tool to compare 2D gel images over the Internet is the Flicker program, which was developed by Lemkin and colleagues at the National Cancer Institute (http://www-lecb.ncifcrf.gov/flicker/). Flicker uses many of the same approaches to the evaluation and matching of gels described earlier. An important feature of Flicker is that it permits the user to compare gel images from different sources on a web browser. This makes possible not only the facile comparison of images from different databases, but also the comparison of one's own 2D gel images with images from different databases.

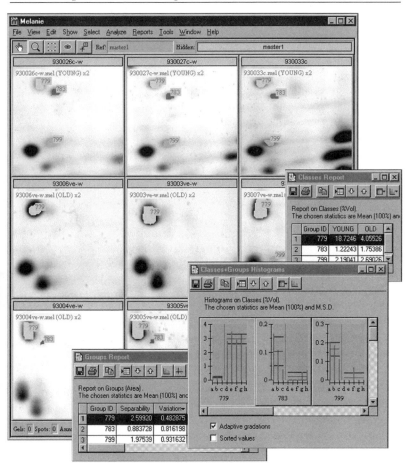

Fig. 2. Quantitation and comparison of spot intensities on multiple 2D gels with Melanie analysis software.

The use of 2D gels is a powerful approach to protein profiling and it is unique in providing a visual-image basis for proteome comparisons. However, there is one major drawback to this approach: staining of 2D gels only detects the more abundant proteins in a sample. There is approximately a million-fold range of protein expression in cells, whereas gel staining is limited by about a hundred-fold dynamic range. It is possible to enhance detection of low-abundance proteins by loading more protein for analysis, but abundant proteins eventually overwhelm many of the features on the gel. A related problem is that many proteins exist in multiply modified forms, which may display different isoelectric points and are thus separated on 2D gels. For less abundant proteins, spreading out into multiple spots can lower detectability by staining. Finally, identification of very weakly stained (and thus low-abundance) proteins by in-gel digestion and MS can be hampered by poor recovery of peptides from the digestion and the gel. As noted in Chapter 5, recovery of peptides from in-gel digestions is usually less than quantitative and is frequently less than 60%. These drawbacks to 2D gel protein profiling all stem from the limited dynamic range of 2D gel staining for protein detection. Although staining and visualization methods are continuing to evolve and improve, this problem may ultimately limit 2D gels to analysis of relatively abundant proteins. This is adequate for many circumstances, however, and 2D gel-based proteome profiling will continue to be a valuable, widely used technique.

12.3. Comparative Proteomics with LC-MS and Isotope Tags

The LC-MS approach to proteome comparisons is conceptually the opposite of the 2D gel approach. Whereas the 2D gel approach separates proteins and begins with an image comparison, the LC-MS approach separates peptides and ends with data mining to assess differences between samples. Here's the LC-MS approach in a nutshell. Two protein samples are treated with reagents to "tag" them. The tags are chemically identical, except that one contains heavy isotopes and the other contains light isotopes. The samples are digested and the peptides are analyzed by LC-MS-MS. Analysis of the MS-MS data (e.g., with Sequest) allows identification of the proteins present. Examination of the full-scan spectra corresponding to each MS-MS scan then allows measurement of the ratio of the light- and heavy-isotope tagged peptides. This ratio corresponds to the ratio of that protein in the two samples. This approach provides not an absolute quantitation of proteins, but rather a relative quantitation of the level of a particular protein in two samples. This approach was first applied to analyzing differences in proteomes by Gygi and Aebersold. We will examine their approach in the following paragraphs, and also consider some possible variants on this approach.

Perhaps the best place to start is with the isotope-labeled tags. The use of isotopic tagging is a variation of the technique known as "stable isotope dilution." To understand why they are used, let's recall that stable isotopes are forms of elements that vary in the number of neutrons in their nuclei, yet are not radioactive. For example, hydrogen has no neutrons, whereas its less abundant isotopomer, deuterium, has one. Thus, hydrogen (^1H) has a mass of one and deuterium (^2H) has a mass of two. Other frequently used stable isotopes are ^{13}C (one amu heavier than ^{12}C), ^{15}N (one amu heavier than ^{14}N), and ^{18}O (two amu heavier than ^{16}O). Compounds labeled with deuterium atoms in place of some of their hydrogen atoms (referred to as "deuterated") have greater molecular mass because each deuterium confers an extra unit of mass. Thus, a compound with eight deuteriums has a mass 8 amu higher than the same unlabeled compound. However, the two compounds will have essentially identical chemical properties, at least in the context of the analytical techniques we are considering. This means that two otherwise identical peptides tagged with an unlabeled and a deuterated reagent will exhibit identical chromatography and display essentially identical ionization and fragmentation in MS. However, the MS instrument distinguishes them as separate species because of their different m/z values. These features make stable isotope-labeled tags ideal agents for labeling, tracking, and quantifying the same peptide in two different samples.

Let's apply stable isotope labeling to the analysis of a particular peptide that is present in two samples. Our hypothetical sample A has 100 pmol of the peptide, whereas sample B has 50 pmol. We treat sample A with a reagent that adds a chemical tag (to the N-terminus, for example) and sample B with a d_{10} (deuterium-labeled) tag (**Fig. 3**). The samples then are mixed and analyzed by LC-MS. Because the unlabeled tagged peptide (from sample A) and the d_{10}-tagged peptide (from sample B) exhibit virtually identical chemical behavior, they elute together from the HPLC column and enter the ESI source at the same time. A full-scan spectrum (**Fig. 3**) indicates signals for both tagged versions. The instrument records a

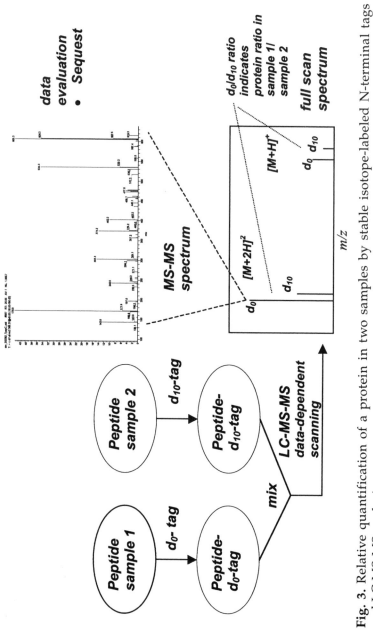

Fig. 3. Relative quantification of a protein in two samples by stable isotope-labeled N-terminal tags and LC-MS-MS analysis.

full-scan spectrum that records the singly and doubly charged ions for the d_0- (unlabeled) and d_{10}-tagged peptides. These are selected and subjected to MS-MS. The MS-MS spectra are essentially identical (except for expected mass differences owing to the difference between the d_0 and d_{10} tag masses), which shows that these two precursor ions in the full-scan spectrum represent the same peptide. Moreover, the MS-MS spectra can be analyzed with Sequest to establish the protein from which they originated. Moreover, the ratio of intensities for the d_0- and d_{10}-tagged peptides ions indicates their ratio in the original samples A and B. In other words, the intensity of the doubly charged ion for the d_0-tagged peptide is twice that for the d_{10}-tagged peptide. This reflects the presence of twice the amount of the peptide in sample A compared to sample B.

Now that we have established how isotope tagging can help us quantify peptides by LC-MS-MS, lets take a closer look at the application of this approach by Gygi and Aebersold. Remember, our "real world" problem is comparative quantification of many proteins between two samples. We face the problems of analyzing a complex protein mixture that can give rise to an even more complex peptide mixture. Each protein may yield many peptides upon tryptic digestion, but we really only need to generate tagged derivatives of one or two representative peptides from each of the proteins to identify them and to provide a basis for measuring relative amounts. The Gygi and Aebersold approach deals with this problem by employing an innovative, multifunctional tagging reagent (**Fig. 4**). The reagent is called an "isotope-coded affinity tag" (ICAT). The reagent has three parts. The first is a thiol-reactive iodoacetamide functional group. This allows the tag to covalently label free cysteinyl thiols in proteins. The second feature is a linker, which may contain either hydrogens (unlabeled, d_0) or deuteriums (labeled, d_8). The third feature is a biotin moiety, which confers high affinity for avidin.

The procedure for the analysis is summarized in **Fig. 5**. Protein sample A is treated with the light d_0-ICAT reagent, whereas sample B is treated with the heavy d_8-ICAT reagent. The reagents label one or more cysteinyl thiols on the proteins. The samples then are combined and digested together with trypsin to generate a very complex digest containing a relatively small proportion of peptides with ICAT tags. The entire mixture is then applied to a column of avidin beads and

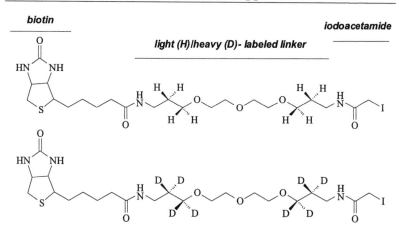

Fig. 4. Thiol-reactive ICAT reagents.

the ICAT-tagged peptides bind tightly through their biotin moieties. The majority of the peptides in the combined sample are then washed away. What remains on the avidin beads are ICAT-tagged peptides from both samples A and B. Thus, the initially very complex tryptic digest has been simplified considerably to a group of bound ICAT-tagged peptides that serve as "representatives" of the proteins from which they originated. The ICAT-tagged peptides are then eluted from the column and analyzed by LC-MS-MS with data-dependent scanning. The analysis of these data is now essentially identical to that illustrated for the simple sample of two peptides in **Fig. 3**. A Sequest analysis of the MS-MS data (with correction of the cysteine residue mass for the presence of the ICAT tag) establishes the peptide and protein sequences that correspond the peptides analyzed. Thus, the ICAT-tagged peptides yield sequence information that permits identification of the proteins from which they originated. Examination of the full scan that corresponds to each MS-MS scan reveals the precursor ions bearing the d_0- and d_8-ICAT tags. The tagged peptides are carried through the entire analysis in proportions that matched those of the proteins from which they originated. These proportions are indicated by the ratio of the d_0- to d_8-ICAT-tagged peptide in the full-scan spectrum. This ratio thus indicates the ratio of the corresponding protein in sample A to that same protein in sample B.

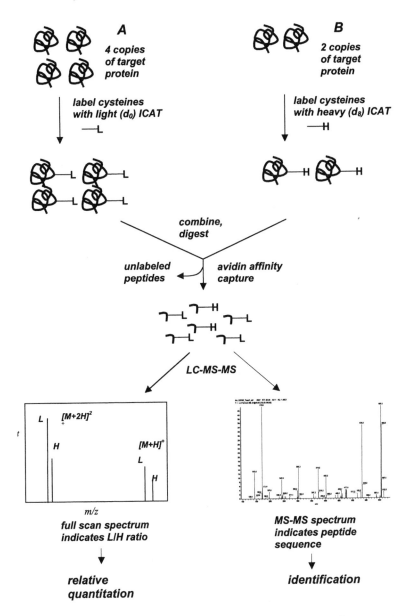

Fig. 5. Schematic representation of relative quantitation of protein in two samples with thiol-reactive ICAT reagents and LC-MS-MS.

For example, analysis of yeast extracts yielded two ICAT-tagged peptides HHIPFYEVDLC*DR and DC*VTLK (the * indicates the ICAT-modified cysteine residue), which both mapped to the protein GAL10. Comparison of the levels of d_0- and d_8-ICAT-HHIPFYEVDLC*DR thus indicates the relative levels of the protein GAL10 in the two samples. This is illustrated by the comparison of proteomes of untreated yeast and yeast treated with ethanol or galactose, which induces significant changes in the levels of many enzymes of intermediary metabolism. Treatment of yeast with galactose and ethanol yielded two samples that were compared by ICAT LC-MS-MS. The ethanol-treated samples were labeled with the d_0-ICAT and the galactose-treated samples were treated with the d_8-ICAT. The ratio of the d_0- to d_8-ICAT-tagged HHIPFYEVDLC*DR and the d_0- to d_8-ICAT-tagged DC*VTLK was 1:>200, which indicated a greater than 200-fold elevation in GAL10 in galactose-treated yeast compared to ethanol-treated yeast.

In general, one to three representative peptides from each protein are analyzed and detected by the ICAT method. The detection of multiple peptides from a protein increases confidence in the assignment of protein identity. Moreover, multiple measurements of d_0/d_8 ICAT peptide ratios increase the accuracy of measurement of the relative levels of that protein in the two samples.

The ultimate expression of the ICAT approach is the combination of isotope tagging with multidimensional peptide separations prior to LC-MS-MS. As discussed in the previous chapter, the use of multidimensional protein and peptide separations combined with LC-MS-MS enhances the detection of relatively low-abundance proteins by "spreading out" the peptide mixture. This provides the MS instrument the opportunity to obtain MS-MS spectra on the greatest number of peptides in the sample. Use of multidimensional peptide separations together with isotope tagging should provide the greatest opportunity to compare changes in expression of low-abundance proteins.

The ICAT approach to proteome comparisons certainly offers some advantages over the 2D gel/MALDI-TOF-based approach. First, the use of LC-MS-MS offers more definitive identification of proteins from complex mixtures than does MALDI-TOF. Second, LC-MS-MS, particularly with multidimensional peptide separations, offers enhanced detection of low-abundance proteins compared to 2D gel analyses, which are limited by the poor dynamic range for protein staining.

Nevertheless there are some limitations of the ICAT technique. First, some proteins either do not contain cysteine residues or else they contain cysteines that are not accessible to the ICAT reagent under the conditions used for tagging. These will not be detected by the ICAT approach. Second, the ICAT approach is essentially a tool for comparing levels of protein expression in two samples. Because only peptides containing ICAT-reactive cysteines are detected in these analyses, most peptides from the proteins are "thrown away" in the avidin bead wash step. With these peptides goes much of the information about changes in protein modifications (e.g., phosphorylation) that may account for changes in the function of that protein between two samples. Unless the modification happens to occur on a cysteine-containing, ICAT-reactive peptide, it will not be detected.

Further variations of the isotope-tagging approach are likely to emerge in the near future. The need for quantitative comparisons of proteomes will become increasingly important in understanding cellular biochemistry. The generic approach is to tag the peptides in two samples with differently labeled tags, then analyze the sample and compare the levels of the differently tagged versions of each peptide. Although the ICAT approach is directed at tagging thiols, it is possible to tag other functional groups in peptides, such as N-terminal amines. This would sacrifice the strategy of greatly simplifying a complex peptide mixture and would certainly necessitate modification of the ICAT approach described earlier. Creative application of isotope-tagging strategies certainly holds great promise for quantitative proteomics.

Suggested Reading

Binz, P. A., Muller, M., Walther, D., Bienvenut, W. V., Gras, R., Hoogland, C., et al. (1999) A molecular scanner to automate proteomic research and to display proteome images. *Anal. Chem.* **71,** 4981–4988.

Gygi, S. P., Rist, B., Gerber, S. A., Turecek, F., Gelb, M. H., and Aebersold, R. (1999) Quantitative analysis of complex protein mixtures using isotope-coded affinity tags. *Nat. Biotechnol.* **17,** 994–999.

Lemkin, P. F. (1997) Comparing two-dimensional electrophoretic gel images across the Internet. *Electrophoresis* **18,** 461–470.

Wilkins, M. R., Gasteiger, E., Bairoch, A., Sanchez, J. C., Williams, K. L., Appel, R. D., and Hochstrasser, D. F. (1999) Protein identification and analysis tools in the ExPASy server. *Methods Mol. Biol.* **112,** 531–552.

13 Identifying Protein–Protein Interactions and Protein Complexes

13.1. "Nothing Propinks Like Propinquity"

Propinquity is a seldom-used noun meaning contact, closeness, or kinship. The previous quote is a political truism testifying to the importance of close personal contact in achieving political success. Proteins are a lot like politicians in that respect, because in most cellular biochemistry, as in legislative politics, teamwork is required.

Proteins "work together" by actually binding to form multicomponent complexes that carry out specific functions. These functional units can be as simple as dimeric transcription-factor complexes or as complex as the 30-plus component systems that form ribosomes. Biochemists have come to appreciate that essentially all proteins bind to or interact with at least one other protein. The discovery that proteins in higher organisms (e.g., human and mouse) contain higher numbers of functional domains suggests that many of these proteins have multiple associations. Understanding how protein complexes work is essential to understanding how cells work as systems.

The first step in understanding these systems, however, is to identify the components. As investigators search for the functions of many newly discovered genes, a key clue is the association of the corresponding proteins with other proteins of known function. For example, many protein kinase signaling complexes involve association of a kinase, a phosphatase, and regulatory proteins together with

From: *Introduction to Proteomics: Tools for the New Biology*
By: D. C. Liebler © Humana Press, Inc., Totowa, NJ

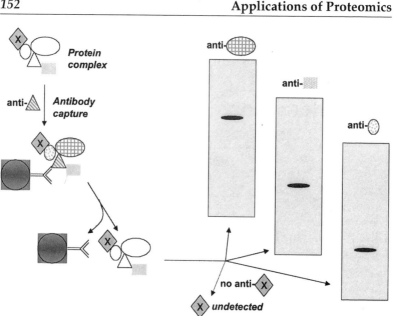

Fig. 1. Dissection of a multiprotein complex by immunoprecipitation and Western-blot analysis.

scaffolding proteins. Although the basic biochemical functions of the kinases and phosphatases could be ascertained by identifying their catalytic domains, the involvement of the accessory proteins in a functional kinase signaling complex would come primarily from a demonstrated association of these proteins.

13.2. Identifying Protein–Protein Interactions

The association of proteins with each other in cellular systems has come primarily from two types of experiments. The first involves the immunoprecipitation of a protein of interest, together with any associated proteins (**Fig. 1**). The proteins then are analyzed by 1D-SDS-PAGE, electrophoretically transferred to a membrane, and the membrane is probed with antibodies suspected as partners of the target protein. Of course, this approach requires that one have antibodies to these proteins and that one be a good guesser. Nevertheless, these antibody

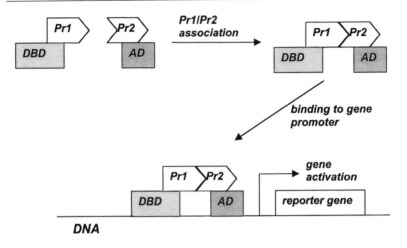

Fig. 2. Schematic representation of the yeast two-hybrid approach to detecting protein–protein interactions.

"pull-down" experiments are very useful tools to confirm suspected protein-protein interactions. Of course, the approach precludes the detection of unanticipated members of multiprotein complexes. For example, in **Fig. 1**, no antibody to the protein marked "X" is available and it is not detected, even though it is present in the complex. There are variants of this general approach, as will be described below. However, the key limitation of this approach is that one can only detect what one sets out to look for in these experiments.

The second major approach is the yeast two-hybrid system (**Fig. 2**). In this approach, detection of the interaction between two proteins is done indirectly. Each of the genes that code for the two proteins of interest (Pr1 and Pr2 in **Fig. 2**) is fused to a transcription factor and then the pair of hybrid genes is expressed in yeast. The transcription-factor components (a DNA-binding domain [DBD] and an activation domain [AD] in **Fig. 2**) encoded by the two different hybrids will activate a reporter gene in the yeast, but only if they become associated with each other to form an active transcription factor. This only happens when the two gene products of interest interact with each other to form a complex. Thus, when the two hybrid proteins of interest form a complex, the transcription-factor pieces are also brought together, the reporter gene is activated, and a signal is detected. This is a powerful assay that has done much to help establish protein-protein interactions for proteins from a variety of species. Because the method of detection is indirect, there are potential confounding factors that can confuse interpretation of the results. These include: 1) failure of some of the hybrid gene products to achieve nuclear localization, 2) interaction of the hybrid gene products with other proteins to prevent activation of the transcription factor components, and 3) the difficulty of expressing some gene products as hybrids in yeast.

13.3. MS Analysis of Protein–Protein Interactions and Complexes: The Basic Approach

Application of the tools of MS-based proteomic analysis offers a new way to identify the components of multiprotein complexes. The generic approach is relatively simple and is described in **Fig. 3**. We begin with a protein of interest (Protein 1), which interacts with unknown protein partners. We prepare cell lysate and then add an antibody to Protein 1 to immunoprecipitate it and any of its partners. This complex can be analyzed in either of two ways.

One approach is to resolve them on a 1D-SDS-PAGE gel, stain and select the protein bands, digest them, and analyze by MALDI-TOF. The proteins can then be identified from the MS data with the aid of peptide mass fingerprinting algorithms (*see* Chapter 7). This is depicted in the upper part of **Fig. 3**. One can also use LC-MS-MS to obtain MS-MS spectra for peptides from these gel bands and then make identifications with database correlation algorithms, such as Sequest. A potential problem with the use of the SDS-PAGE step is that it often results in loss of protein, owing both to incomplete in-gel digestion and to incomplete recovery of the peptides from the gel. This can complicate detection of low-abundance proteins in a mixture. On the other hand, the use of a protein-resolving step is often necessary to increase the effectiveness of protein identification by MALDI-TOF MS and peptide mass fingerprinting (*see* below).

The other approach to identify the proteins present in the immunoprecipitate is to digest them directly (without first separating them from each other) and then to analyze the peptide-digest mixture by MALDI-TOF MS or by LC-MS-MS. This is referred to as "shotgun"

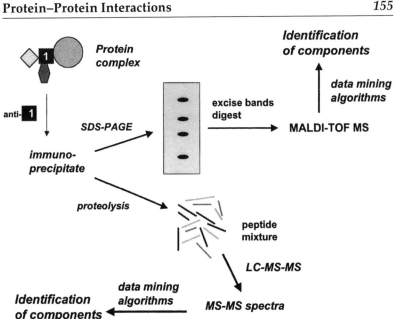

Fig. 3. Dissection of a multiprotein complex by immunoprecipitation and 1D-SDS-PAGE/MALDI-TOF (*top*) or "shotgun" identification by LC-MS-MS (*bottom*).

analysis (in analogy to the DNA sequencing strategy) and it works very well. The approach is depicted in the lower part of **Fig. 3**. Direct MALDI-TOF MS analysis of the peptide mixture would be complicated by the presence of peptides from the several different proteins in the complex, including those derived from the antibody. (The antibody can be eliminated from the analysis, as discussed below.) If the complex contained three or fewer proteins, identification of these by direct MALDI-TOF analysis would be relatively straightforward. With larger numbers of proteins present, the complexity of the MALDI-TOF spectra would make identification increasingly difficult.

These complications make MALDI-TOF less applicable to shotgun analysis of peptide mixtures than LC-MS-MS, which is much better suited to the analysis of more complex peptide mixtures. Identification of proteins would be based on analysis of the MS-MS spectra of the peptides with a sequence correlation algorithm such as Sequest.

Whereas the presence of peptides from multiple proteins can generate exceedingly complicated MALDI-TOF spectra, LC-MS-MS acquires spectra from individual peptides, which then can be analyzed individually. For moderately complex protein mixtures (e.g., 2–5 proteins), a simple LC-MS-MS analysis with data reduction aided by Sequest can identify the partners. Indeed, this approach has been employed by several groups to characterize relatively small multiprotein complexes. However, for more complex mixtures, the number of peptides from each protein that are actually subjected to MS-MS may actually diminish. In other words, with many more peptides coming off the LC column, the instrument may be busy obtaining an MS-MS spectrum of one peptide ion while another "sneaks" by unnoticed. This diminishes sequence coverage (i.e., the number of peptides from each protein identified), which in turn diminishes our confidence in the identifications made. To increase the degree of sequence coverage, multidimensional peptide separations can be employed (*see* Chapter 11). Link and colleagues used in-line ion exchange and RP LC with MS-MS to analyze a 78 subunit yeast ribosomal complex. Use of the multidimensional peptide separation in line with MS-MS significantly increased the number of proteins identified as well as the sequence coverage for each protein.

The foregoing sections indicate that one may use either relatively simple (e.g., MALDI-TOF) or relatively complex (tandem LC-ESI-MS-MS) approaches to MS identification of proteins in an immunoprecipitated sample. Which approach works best depends largely on the amount of protein to be characterized and the numbers of proteins in the complex. Once the MS methods are established and in place in a laboratory, this end of the analysis is relatively straightforward. The real challenge in mapping protein-protein interactions lies in obtaining protein samples that actually represent biologically relevant protein complexes or protein-protein interactions. We have used immunoprecipitation as an example, but there are other means of isolating complexes. The following sections describe approaches to isolating these complexes.

13.4. Immunoprecipitations

Perhaps the most widely used approach to isolating multiprotein complexes is to immunoprecipitate them with an antibody to one of the

components. The generic example outlined earlier used immunoprecipitation to isolate a complex. Let's consider some of the imperatives
for successful application of the approach. First of these is obtaining
a suitable antibody. The antibody should display specificity for the
protein target of interest. In addition, the antibody should be capable
of immunoprecipitating both the target protein alone and when it is
bound to its complex partners. Not all antibodies are well-suited to
immunoprecipation and the antibody thus should be tested for the
ability to immunoprecipitate its target protein.

Another potential complication is that the antibody may successfully
immunoprecipitate its target protein, but not when other interacting
proteins are present. This may be owing either to lack of sufficient
antibody specificity (i.e., the antibody reacts with other proteins) or
to binding of other proteins to the antibody-recognition site on the
target protein. This could occur if a partner of the target protein in the
complex "covers up" the antibody-binding site.

The antibody is a useful tool to isolate the complex between the
target protein and its partners. However, once the complex is in
hand, the antibody can complicate analysis. Regardless of whether
MALDI-TOF or LC-MS-MS is used for analysis of the peptides from
the complex, the sample will also contain significant amounts of
peptides derived from the antibody. These antibody-derived peptides
can complicate analysis and reduce sensitivity for identification of
true members of the target protein complex. Perhaps the most effective
means of circumventing this problem is to use an antibody that is
covalently linked to an insoluble bead. There are commercially available kits that make it easy to generate immobilized antibodies. With
these bead-linked antibodies, immunoprecipitations are followed by
brief treatment with a denaturant (e.g., 1 M acetic acid), which releases
the bound protein from the bead-linked antibody. The antibody is
recovered by centrifugation or filtration and capture of the beads.
The eluted proteins then are subjected to digestion and MS analysis
without the presence of interfering antibody-derived peptides.

Once putative partners of the target protein are identified, some
means of confirming the findings of the immunoprecipitation experiment is desirable. We would like to get some complementary evidence
that the complexation we observed is not some artifact of the immunoprecipitation experiment. Certainly, the identification of proteins

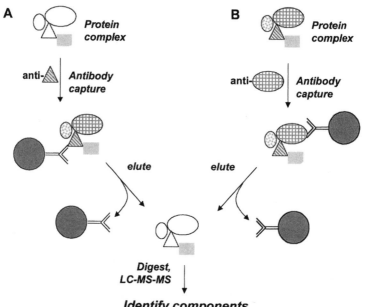

Fig. 4. Detection of protein complex members by immunoprecipitation with antibody to one complex member **(A)**, followed by a separate immunoprecipitation with another putative member of the complex **(B)**.

with known and related functions, such as a kinase together with a phosphatase and a scaffolding protein, makes sense. However, we can attempt to better document the association of our target protein with one of its putative partners. By using an antibody to one of the associated proteins for another immunoprecipitation experiment, we can see whether we identify the original target protein as a partner in the complex (e.g., compare the results of experiments A and B in **Fig. 4**). A series of immunoprecipitations of this type can be used to confirm the associations identified in the initial experiment.

13.5. Bait and Reverse Bait

An alternative to the use of antibodies for capturing protein complexes is to use the "bait" approach, in which the target protein of interest is immobilized on a solid support (**Fig. 5A**). There are several

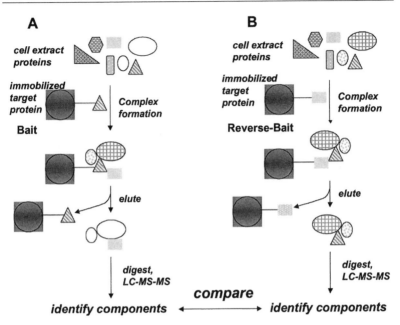

Fig. 5. Schematic representation of the "bait" (**A**) and "reverse-bait" (**B**) approach to identify members of a multiprotein complex.

ways to link the target protein to a bead or similar support. Covalent linkage can be achieved by incubation of the protein with an activated support, such as epoxyalkylSepharose, which reacts covalently with nucleophilic amine or thiol groups on the protein. Alternatively, recombinant proteins containing His-tag or FLAG-tag sequences can be generated. These then associate tightly with immobilized nickel resins or immobilized anti-FLAG antibodies. The bead-linked protein is then incubated with a cell lysate or similar extract, which contains putative partners (**Fig. 5**). The partner proteins then associate with the immobilized target protein to form the multiprotein complex. The immobilized complex is then harvested by centrifugation or filtration and the associated proteins are dissociated from the complex, digested, and analyzed. The considerations for choosing a particular MS analytical method are the same as those described previously for analyzing immunoprecipitated proteins.

There are two advantages of the "bait" approach over immunoprecipitation experiments. First, there is no antibody present in the captured complex to complicate the analysis. Second, one need not be concerned about whether an antibody recognizes the appropriate epitope on the target protein in a complex. Of course, it is possible that the linkage of the target protein may interfere with a protein interaction that would otherwise occur in vivo. For example, an interaction of the N-terminal domain of the target protein with another protein could be disrupted by immobilization of the target protein through the N-terminus. However, this concern can be mitigated somewhat by control experiments described below. Another disadvantage of the bait approach relative to the immunoprecipitation approach is that one must generate or obtain the immobilized target protein. Depending on the available resources, this may be more expensive, difficult, or time-consuming than simply raising or buying an antibody.

Once one has identified putative partners of the target protein using the bait approach, confirmation of the interaction can be obtained by performing a "reverse bait" experiment (**Fig. 5B**). To do this we examine the list of putative partners identified in the bait experiment. We then select one and prepare an immobilized version of that protein. We then perform the same type of experiment in the same system. Identification of the associated proteins found in this experiment should reveal the original target protein, as well as others found in the original experiment. This provides confirmation of the association of these proteins under the experimental conditions. One may also find associated proteins not found in the original experiment, which can provide new leads for mapping other members of a network. This extension of the reverse-bait approach is discussed later in this chapter.

13.6. Multiprotein-Nucleic Acid Complexes

An important class of protein-protein interactions is that of proteins interacting with specific nucleic acid sequences, such as in the promoter elements of genes. These interactions involve not only interactions between several proteins associated with transcription and repair, but also critical interactions with defined nucleotide sequences. The most common means of characterizing these interactions is the electrophoretic mobility shift assay (EMSA), which is illustrated in

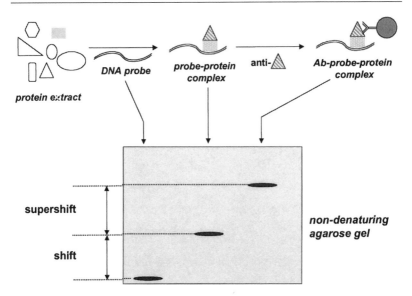

Fig. 6. Schematic representation of the "gel shift" and "supershift" assays to detect proteins that interact with specific DNA sequences.

Fig. 6. An oligonucleotide probe containing the sequence of interest is labeled with ^{32}P and then incubated with a cell or nuclear lysate containing putative interacting proteins. An extract from the mixture is then subjected to agarose gel electrophoresis under nondenaturing conditions. Oligonucleotide probe that is not complexed with an interacting protein(s) migrates through the gel easily, whereas labeled oligonucleotide that is complexed with protein migrates more slowly. The difference in migration is referred to as the gel "shift" and indicates (it is hoped) a specific association of one or more proteins with that sequence element. To identify the interacting proteins, one may incubate the complex with an antibody to the suspected proteins prior to performing the electrophoresis. If an antibody recognizes and binds to a protein in the complex, the antibody-bound complex migrates through the gel even more slowly. This additional shift is termed a "supershift" and provides identification of at lease one member of the complex. Of course, the limitation of this approach is that antibody binding does not necessarily amount to definitive

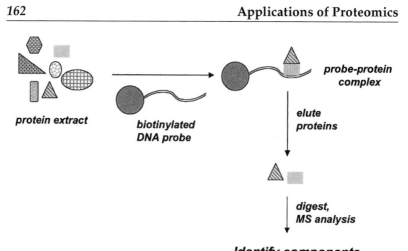

Fig. 7. "Bait" approach to detection of DNA-interacting proteins with a biotinylated-DNA probe.

identification of the protein in the complex. More importantly, one must guess which antibody to use and thus this approach precludes discovery of novel protein components of the complex.

Analytical proteomics can be applied to this problem in two ways. First, the bands that display a gel shift or a supershift can be excised and the proteins can be digested and analyzed by MS. However, the amounts of protein present in these samples is typically rather small (due to the sensitivity of detection of ^{32}P by autoradiography) and this may make identification difficult, unless the experiment is scaled-up or multiple replicate samples are combined.

A second approach to identifying oligonucleotide-interacting proteins is to use a variation of the bait experiment described earlier. The "bait" in this case can be an oligonucleotide that is immobilized on a solid support (**Fig. 7**). For example, a biotinylated oligonucleotide can be used to capture nucleic acid-interacting proteins and their associated proteins. The entire complex then can be captured with an avidin-coated bead; nonspecifically associated proteins can be removed by washing; and the specifically associated proteins then eluted, digested, and analyzed. The principal difficulty with this approach is in capturing proteins with a high binding specificity for the

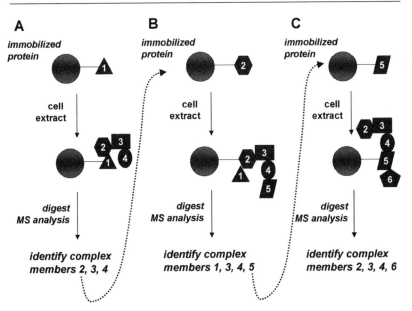

Fig. 8. Mapping a protein-interaction network with a series of linked "bait" and "reverse-bait" experiments.

sequence element being studied. This approach is currently in development in several laboratories and should eventually supersede EMSA techniques for characterizing nucleic acid-interacting proteins.

13.7. Protein Network Mapping

If we accept the proposition that essentially all proteins bind to at least one other protein in cells, then it follows that proteins form networks of association. This has been elegantly demonstrated by Fields and colleagues in their systematic application of the yeast two-hybrid approach to mapping protein-interaction networks in yeast. An alternative approach to the yeast two-hybrid assay for mapping protein-interaction networks is an extended application of the bait and reverse-bait experiments described earlier. This approach to protein network mapping is described in **Fig. 8**. We start with our initial target protein, Protein 1, which is immobilized on a bead support. Incubation of this "bait" with a cell lysate and MS analysis of the recovered proteins reveals partners Protein 2, Protein 3, and Protein 4. This is followed with a reverse-bait experiment with immobilized Protein 2, which reveals associated Protein 1, Protein 3, Protein 4, and a new protein, which is designated Protein 5. Next, an immobilized Protein 5 is prepared and used as bait for another experiment in the same system. MS analysis of proteins associated with Protein 5 reveals Protein 2, Protein 3, Protein 4, and another new protein, which is designated Protein 6. This cycle of analyses may be continued indefinitely. For each finding of a protein association, a reverse-bait experiment can be performed to confirm the finding.

The net result of these bait and reverse-bait experiments is to map a network of protein-protein associations, which may indicate functions of these proteins in a systems context. Of course, the approach outlined here would require the ability to generate immobilized proteins for each experiment, which could be rather time-consuming. An alternative is the use of antibodies to perform immunoprecipitation experiments with an overall similar strategy. The advantages and disadvantages of employing antibodies described earlier also apply here. Regardless of the specific technique (bait vs antibody), this general approach offers the clear advantage of definitive identification of the interacting proteins at each step in mapping the network.

Suggested Reading

Craig, T. A., Benson, L. M., Tomlinson, A. J., Veenstra, T. D., Naylor, S., and Kumar, R. (1999) Analysis of transcription complexes and effects of ligands by microelectrospray ionization mass spectrometry. *Nat. Biotechnol.* **17,** 1214–1218.

Honey, S., Schneider, B. L., Schieltz, D. M., Yates, J. R., and Futcher, B. (2001) A novel multiple affinity purification tag and its use in identification of proteins associated with a cyclin-CDK complex. *Nucleic Acids Res.* **29,** E24.

Ng, D. H., Watts, J. D., Aebersold, R., and Johnson, P. (1996) Demonstration of a direct interaction between p56lck and the cytoplasmic domain of CD45 in vitro. *J. Biol. Chem.* **271,** 1295–1300.

Panigrahi, A. K., Gygi, S. P., Ernst, N. L., Igo, R. P., Palazzo, S. S., Schnaufer, A., et al. (2001) Association of two novel proteins, TbMP52 and TbMP48, with the Trypanosoma brucei RNA editing complex. *Mol. Cell Biol.* **21,** 380–389.

Rigaut, G., Shevchenko, A., Rutz, B., Wilm, M., Mann, M., and Seraphin, B. (1999) A generic protein purification method for protein complex characterization and proteome exploration. *Nat. Biotechnol.* **17,** 1030–1032.

Rudiger, A. H., Rudiger, M., Carl, U. D., Chakraborty, T., Roepstorff, P., and Wehland, J. (1999) Affinity mass spectrometry-based approaches for the analysis of protein-protein interaction and complex mixtures of peptide-ligands. *Anal. Biochem.* **275,** 162–170.

Schwikonski, B., Vetz, P. and Fields, S. (2000) A network of protein–protein interactions in yeast. *Nat. Biotechnol.* **18,** 1257–1261.

Yates, J. R. (2000) Mass spectrometry: from genomics to proteomics. *Trends Genet.* **16,** 5–8

14 Mapping Protein Modifications

14.1. Protein Modifications Everywhere

An emerging truism of proteomics is that most proteins are present in living systems in multiply modified forms. In reviewing the "life cycle" of a protein in Chapter 2, we considered the formation of polypeptides on ribosomes, their posttranslational cleavage, their modification by endogenous and exogenous agents, the accumulation of oxidative damage, and their eventual degradation. All of these events involve distinct modifications to protein structures. The occurrence of modifications at multiple sites on some proteins adds to the complexity of the situation. Many of the techniques of protein biochemistry used over the past 50 years have allowed us to determine whether a protein is modified. In most cases, the determination tells us that the protein is modified, but does not tell us where it is modified. Knowing this is important, because the same modification at different sites may have different consequences.

In much recent work in biochemistry and cell biology, investigators have used combinations of tools other than MS to map protein modifications. Perhaps the two most widely used approaches are antibodies and site-directed mutagenesis. The mapping of phosphorylation sites in proteins provides a useful example of how these two techniques are used. Monoclonal antibodies (MAbs) directed against phosphoserine/phosphothreonine or phosphotyrosine can be used to map these residues to intact proteins or cleaved peptides. Site-directed

From: *Introduction to Proteomics: Tools for the New Biology*
By: D. C. Liebler © Humana Press, Inc., Totowa, NJ

mutagenesis allows the investigator to systematically "knock out" serine, threonine, or tyrosine residues thought to be phosphorylated in the system under study. Western-blot analysis of these proteins or their peptide fragments with the antibodies can confirm whether phosphorylation was knocked out by specific amino acid substitutions. This allows the investigator to infer which amino acids are the sites of modification.

There are two problems with this approach. First, one can never be sure whether the amino acid substitutions used in site-directed mutagenesis change some other aspect of the system, such as the association with a kinase, for example. Even subtle structural changes in a kinase phosphorylation motif induced by the substitution may affect phosphorylation at adjacent acceptor sites. This can be particularly troublesome in peptides where mutiple potential phosphorylation targets occur together in close proximity. A second problem is a practical one. It takes tremendous effort to generate the antibodies and mutant proteins to do these types of studies. The issue of antibody specificity must be addressed every time a new protein system is studied. This second issue creates a significant barrier to attempting these studies. Although phosphorylation has been studied extensively in this way, there are many other interesting modifications that may not be as amenable to this approach.

The introduction of MS methods to analyze peptides now offers the best means to characterize protein modifications. The features of MS data that allow us to determine peptide masses and sequences also provide information about modifications on the peptides. Moreover, the identification of specific modifications can be facilitated by some of the MS data mining and software tools we considered in earlier chapters. In this chapter, we will examine how we can combine MS analyses and data mining to map unambiguously and accurately protein modifications at the level of amino acid sequence. These concepts will be developed in the context of mapping protein phosphorylation sites and then extended to mapping of other endogenous modifications as well as exogenous modifications by environmental chemicals.

14.2. The Name of the Game is Coverage

Up to this point, our focus in MS analysis of proteins has been on the identification and relative quantitation of proteins. In many cases, tryptic digestion followed by MS analysis provides data on multiple peptides from a protein. The extent to which the entire protein sequence is represented by MS data is often referred to as "coverage." For example, if we analyze a tryptic digest of a 100 amino acid protein and we obtain MS data on tryptic peptides corresponding to 60 residues, we say that we have 60% sequence coverage. For purposes of simply identifying a protein, this is usually more than enough. Remember, in peptide mass fingerprinting with MALDI-TOF data, matches of as few as 2–3 peptides to database entries is often sufficient to establish the identity of the protein. In practice, this may translate to as little as 10–15% sequence coverage. In LC-MS-MS, good MS-MS spectra of two 6-mer peptides from the 100 amino acid protein can provide definitive identification of a protein. This would amount to only 12% coverage. Thus, limited coverage does not prevent reliable protein identification. The same can be said for quantification of protein expression. With either 2D gels-based image comparisons or LC-MS-MS with stable isotope tags, the identity of the protein being quantified can be established with as little as 5–10% sequence coverage.

The situation is very different when one tries to map protein modifications by MS. We can only detect peptide modifications if we have MS data for the modified peptide. To check a protein for modifications on all possible amino acids, we must have MS data for all the peptides. In other words, we must have 100% sequence coverage. This point is illustrated in **Fig. 1**. If we perform a tryptic digest of this protein and then obtain MS-MS spectra and sequence of peptides 1, 4, and 7, we can certainly identify the protein (**Fig. 1A**). However, phosphorylation occurs in peptides 2 and 8. However, with data only for peptides 1, 4, and 7, we could not map the phosphorylation sites, which occurred on other peptides. If we obtained MS-MS spectra on peptides 2 and 8 (**Fig. 1B**), which contain the phosphoserine residues, we would not only be able to identify the protein, we could deduce the exact sites of phosphorylation on those two peptides (*see* below). It seems unlikely that we would be so lucky with every protein we study. Nevertheless, this example illustrates the importance of coverage in mapping protein modifications. We must rely on coverage or luck. Because we cannot always count on luck, we will have to work to improve coverage. Before we discuss strategies to do that, let's

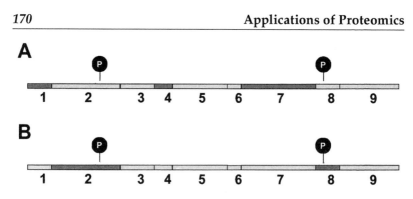

Fig. 1. Schematic representation of the effect of sequence coverage on detection of posttranslational modifications. The dark segments of the proteins represent sequence for which MS data have been obtained. The sites of phosphorylation are indicated on peptides 2 and 8.

consider what information in MS data can help us map modifications to specific amino acid residues.

14.3. Deducing Modifications from MS Data

If we use MALDI-TOF to obtain MS-MS spectra of a mixture of peptides, the data provide accurate mass measurements of the peptide ions. The measured masses reflect the amino acid composition of the peptides, plus the masses of any modifications. Thus, MALDI-TOF MS analysis can tell us which peptides may be present in modified form. For example, MALDI-TOF analysis of a mixture of a phosphorylated peptide and its unphosphorylated counterpart will yield two signals. The one at lower m/z is for the unphosphorylated peptide, whereas the one at an m/z value of 80 units higher corresponds to the phosphorylated peptide.

The combination of MALDI-TOF MS analysis and peptide mass fingerprinting algorithms and software makes it possible to not only identify proteins, but also to identify modified forms. These software tools allow the user to specify common modifications such as phosphorylation as well as unique, user-defined modifications. Thus MS signals that do not correspond to unmodified peptides in a database may be matched to their modified counterparts.

This can be useful for mapping modifications to specific peptides. However, the approach does not unambiguously map modifications to specific amino acids. For example, the VPQLEIVPNpSAEER peptide contains only one plausible site for phosphorylation at the serine residue. Other peptides may contain multiple possible phosphorylation sites. The peptide GQSTSRHK from the human p53 protein contains two serines, both of which are sites of phosphorylation by kinases. The unmodified peptide has an [M+H]$^+$ ion at m/z 900.9760, whereas the monophosphorylated form has an [M+H]$^+$ ion at m/z 980.9558. Unfortunately, this number does not tell us which of the two serines is phosphorylated. We might be able to infer the *probable* site of phosphorylation if we knew the preferred phosphorylation motif of the kinase that phosphorylated the protein. Often, we do not have that information. Even if we did, we could only make an inference, not a definitive identification. To do this, we must obtain an MS-MS spectrum of the peptide ion.

LC-MS-MS provides MS-MS spectra of peptides that allow us to infer not only sequence information, but also the sequence location of modifications. For example, an MS-MS spectrum of the phospho-peptide VPQLEIVPNpSAEER from bovine casein is shown in **Fig. 2**. The mass of the doubly charged ion (m/z 831.2) is 40 units above that of that expected for the unmodified peptide (m/z 791.4). This confirms the presence of a phosphorylation. The spectrum contains b- and y-ion series ions, which provide the sequence information. The spectrum shows a shift in the y-ion series beginning with the y_5 ion, which appears at 80 m/z units above that expected for the corresponding unphosphorylated peptide (i.e., m/z 671.2 for the phosphorylated form vs m/z 591.6 for the unphosphorylated form). Moreover, signals for the y_7, y_8, y_9, and y_{11} ions appear at 80 m/z above the corresponding product ions for the unmodified peptide. (The y_6, y_{10}, y_{12}, and y_{13} ions do not appear in the spectrum.) Only one b-ion (b13) containing the phosphoserine residue appears in the spectrum, but its m/z is shifted by 80 amu to reflect the presence of the phosphorylation. The alterations in the b- and y-ion series confirm the sequence position of the modified residue. Another interesting feature of the MS-MS spectrum is the strong product ion at m/z 782.1. This ion results from loss of phosphoric acid (98 da) from the serine as a neutral fragment (**Fig. 2**). (Remember, a neutral loss of phosphoric acid (98 da) from a doubly charged ion gives a signal 49 units below the doubly charged precorsor m/z. This is why the loss from the doubly

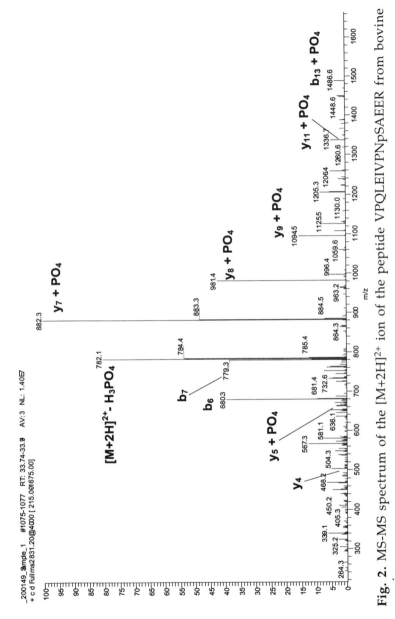

Fig. 2. MS-MS spectrum of the $[M+2H]^{2+}$ ion of the peptide VPQLEIVPNpSAEER from bovine casein.

charged phosphopeptide at m/z 831.2 in **Fig. 2** yields a fragment at m/z 782.1. Loss of the same fragment from a singly charged precursor gives a signal 98 units below the singly charged precursor m/z.) This facile elimination is characteristic of both phosphoserine and phosphothreonine residues in MS-MS. In contrast, phosphotyrosine residues do not readily lose phosphoric acid, as they have no hydrogen alpha to the phosphate to facilitate the elimination reaction. The combination of an altered mass for the $[M+2H]^{2+}$ precursor ion, the neutral loss of 49 units (i.e., phosphoric acid) from the doubly charged ion and the appearance of 80 amu shifts in the b- and y-ions containing the phosphoserine definitively confirm the presence and sequence location of phosphorylation on serine in this peptide.

The criteria we have applied in this example can be applied to map essentially any chemical modification in a protein. LC-MS-MS is superior to MALDI-TOF and peptide mass fingerprinting for this type of work because MS-MS spectra provide both peptide sequence information (b- and y-ions) and other information specific to the modification itself (e.g., neutral losses or productions). We will consider the applicability of these modification-specific spectral features to characterizing other protein modifications later in this chapter.

14.4. Sample Enrichment

It seems clear that once we obtain good quality MS or MS-MS spectra of modified peptides, we can identify the peptide and the site of modification. The biggest problem with mapping modifications is simply obtaining MS or MS-MS spectra of the modified peptides. Of all the copies of any particular protein in a cell, only a small fraction may bear any specific modification. For example, many protein kinase substrates are rapidly phosphorylated and dephosphorylated, such that only a few phosphorylated copies of a protein may be present at a particular time. When we attempt to analyze a protein sample for the modification, most of the peptides in our sample are unmodified. In MALDI-TOF analysis, this will mean that we have much more intense signals for the unmodified than for the modified peptides. For LC-MS-MS analysis, it will mean that the peptide ions corresponding to the unmodified peptides are more intense and are more likely to be selected for MS-MS fragmentation than the ions from the modified peptides.

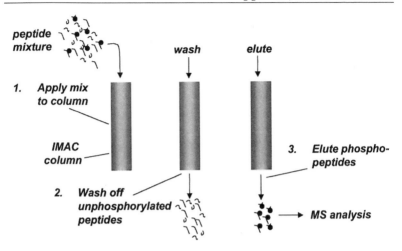

Fig. 3. Use of immobilized metal affinity chromatography (IMAC) to isolate phosphopeptides from a peptide digest.

One obvious solution to this problem is to employ an enrichment strategy to increase the fraction of modified proteins or peptides in the sample to be studied. This can be done at the protein or the peptide level, depending on the nature and the abundance of the modification. Although most modifications are small relative to entire proteins, they may alter some property of the protein. For example, modifications that alter isoelectric points of proteins can affect their migration on 2D gels and the individually modified forms can appear as "spot trains" (*see* Chapter 4). Because peptides are much smaller than proteins, modifications on peptides may more significantly affect their behavior and chemistry. For modified peptides, an enrichment strategy must be directed at some chemical, physical, or immunologic property of the modifying moiety itself. The general approach to this is illustrated in **Fig. 3**. A protein digest containing modified and unmodified peptides is applied to a column containing some immobilized ligand. The unmodified peptides have less affinity for the column and pass through easily, whereas the modified peptides bind more tightly. Washing elutes the unmodified peptides. The modified peptides then are eluted with a solution that disrupts their interaction with the immobilized ligand. Phosphorylated peptides display significant affinity for immobilized metals because of the strong affinity of the anionic phosphate groups for polyvalent metal cations. This property has led to the development of immobilized metal affinity chromatography (IMAC) methods for isolating phosphopeptides from protein digests. Although they can significantly enrich the sample in phosphorylated peptides, we must remember that all phosphopeptides will vary somewhat in their affinities for the IMAC ligands. This makes the use of these columns very tricky, thus necessitating careful refinement of protocols. Another variation on the theme of enrichment uses immobilized antibodies directed against the modifying moiety. For example, antibodies against phosphorylated amino acids could be used to capture phosphopeptides by immunoprecipitation or with immobilized antibody columns. As with IMAC methods, the success of this approach is dependent on the affinity of the antibody for the modified peptide compared to the unmodified peptide. For capture of peptides modified by xenobiotics (*see* below), this may be a viable approach, as such antibodies have been used in analogous enrichment of nucleic acid adducts for subsequent MS analysis. As with antiphospho-amino acid antibodies, the affinity of the antibody for the modified peptides will dictate the degree to which the method enriches the sample. All of these considerations suggest that individual enrichment strategies require careful optimization and attention to detail.

14.5. Mining MS-MS Data for Modifications

As we noted earlier, once we obtain MS-MS spectra of modified peptides, we have a reasonable chance of deducing both the sequence of the peptide and the location of the modification. Even if we devise strategies to enrich samples for modified peptides, the enrichment is not perfect and we still must sort through many MS-MS spectra to determine which correspond to modified peptides. This dilemma is similar to those we face in essentially all LC-MS-MS analyses of peptide mixtures: we have a tremendous amount of data to deal with. Fortunately, we can use familiar data-reduction algorithms and software tools to sift the data for those MS-MS scans that correspond to modified peptides. The Sequest program allows the user to specify a number of common, low molecular-weight modifications that may appear on proteins. For example, the user may specify that serines, threonines, and/or tyrosone residues *may* be phosphorylated in the peptides whose MS-MS spectra are being analyzed. Sequest then performs correlations of the MS-MS data with virtual MS-MS scans generated from database sequences in which these amino acids are either modified or unmodified. For example, an MS-MS scan may display significant Sequest correlation scores to a database sequence that has a serine residue. If the correlation to the phosphoserine peptide sequence is strong, while that for the unphosphorylated sequence is weak, it is likely that the MS-MS spectrum is from the phosphorylated peptide. If inspection of the Sequest-assigned ions in the spectrum verifies the expected shifts in the b- and y-ion series due to phosphorylation, the assignment can be made with confidence. In this way, Sequest can be used to map a variety of simple, low molecular-weight peptide modifications. This approach can work very well as long as: 1) one can anticipate the chemical nature (i.e., the mass) of the modification, 2) the modification results in a change in the MS-MS spectrum, and 3) the mass of the modification is within the limits imposed by Sequest or similar programs.

A second approach to the detection of protein modifications is to analyze the MS-MS data with the SALSA algorithm, which was described in Chapter 10. Many peptide modifications give rise to specific features of MS-MS spectra. For example, phosphorylated serine and threonine residues eliminate phosphoric acid (98 da) in MS-MS (*see* **Fig. 2**). Thus, product ions at 49 and 98 units below doubly and singly charged precursor ions, respectively, are observed in the spectra. Other modifications may yield specific product ions in MS-MS spectra. For example, peptides modified with polycyclic aromatic hydrocarbons fragment with dissociation of the hydrocarbon moiety as an intense product ion. Finally, stable modifications of any amino acid in a peptide sequence will alter the b- and/or y-ion series in the MS-MS spectrum. This is because the modification affects the apparent residue mass of the modified amino acid. Consider the example of the AVAGCAGAR peptide we discussed in Chapter 8. **Fig. 4** shows the MS-MS spectra of unmodified AVAGCAGAR (top) and S-carboxymethyl-AVAGCAGAR (bottom). The y_1–y_4 ions for the two peptides have identical *m/z* values (the y_1 ion is not detected), but the y_5 ions differ. In the unmodified peptide, the y_5 ion CAGAR$^+$ is at *m/z*

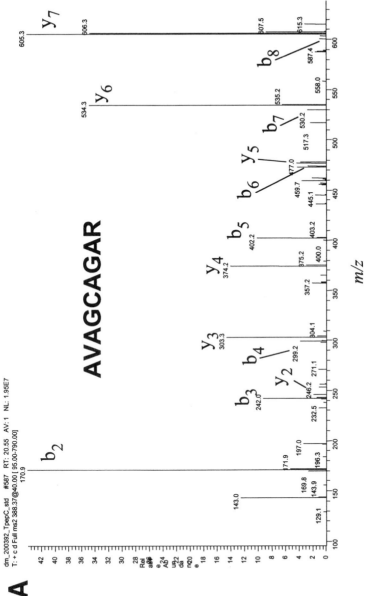

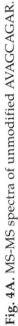

Fig. 4A. MS-MS spectra of unmodified AVAGCAGAR.

177

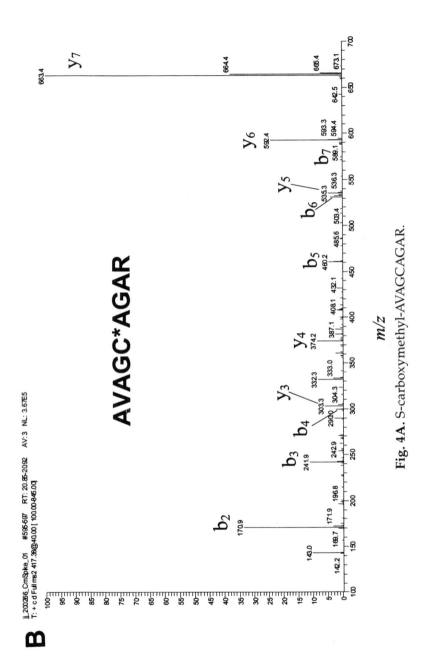

Fig. 4A. S-carboxymethyl-AVAGCAGAR.

477, whereas the y_5 ion from the modified peptide S-carboxymethyl-CAGAR$^+$ is at m/z 535. The mass difference is 58, which corresponds to the carboxymethyl modification. In the modified peptide, the y_5–y_8 ions are all 59 m/z units higher than those in the MS-MS spectrum of the unmodified peptide. The same changes occur in the b-ion series. The b_1–b_4 ions are the same in both peptides, but the b_5–b_8 ions of the modified peptide also fall 58 m/z units above the b_5–b_8 ions in the unmodified peptide.

In Chapter 10, we discussed the ability of the SALSA algorithm to detect MS-MS spectra that displayed a particular series of ions separated by defined values. In this way, an ion-series *pattern* represents a specific amino acid motif. SALSA generates a "virtual ruler" defined by the spacing of ions relative to each other in the b- or y-ion series. This ruler is then held up to the MS-MS scans to detect those spectra with ion series that match the ruler. For the AVAGCAGAR peptide and its variants, we used a "GACGA" ruler corresponding to the central part of the peptide sequence. In the earlier example, the introduction of a modification at the cysteine residue in AVAGCAGAR shifts the y- and b-ion series beginning with the y_5 and b_5 ions, respectively. Consequently, the ruler would match with part, but not all of the y-ion series for the modified peptide (**Fig. 5**). When aligned beginning with the highest observed y-ion (y_7), the y_7, y_6, and y_5 ions match the ruler, but the y_2, y_3, and y_4 ions do not. If we match beginning with the lowest observed y-ion (y_2, not labeled in **Fig. 5**), the y_2–y_4 ions match, but the y_5–y_7 ions do not. Thus, we have a partial match either way. SALSA will assign a significant score to these partially matched MS-MS spectra, but the scores will not be as high as those for the MS-MS spectra of the unmodified peptide. Nevertheless, these partial ion-series matches will allow SALSA to identify MS-MS spectra that correspond to modified peptides. Analysis of the MS-MS spectra will allow us to confirm the peptide sequence and the exact location of the modification. In this way, we can map that modified peptide back to a protein sequence in a database and establish the protein that was modified and the site of modification.

This general approach can be a powerful tool for characterizing proteomes, where protein modifications influence function, protein-protein interactions, and protein turnover. The power of the SALSA algorithm is in its ability to distinguish spectra that display the

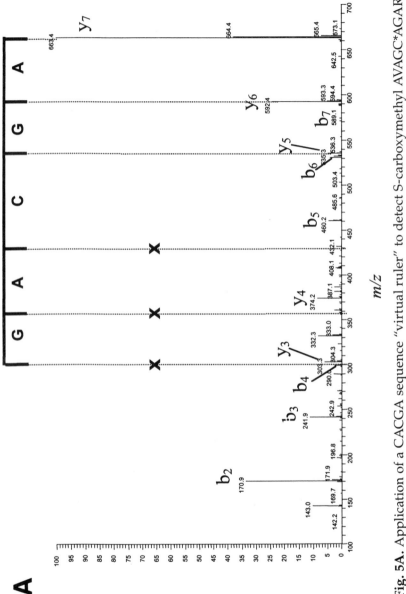

Fig. 5A. Application of a CACGA sequence "virtual ruler" to detect S-carboxymethyl AVAGC*AGAR in high m/z v ions.

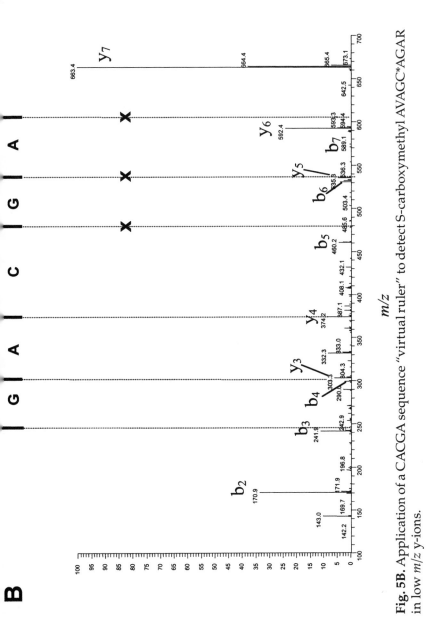

Fig. 5B. Application of a CACGA sequence "virtual ruler" to detect S-carboxymethyl AVAGC*AGAR in low m/z y-ions.

features characteristic of a sequence or a modification or both. We must remember, however, that SALSA cannot identify modified peptides unless our MS analysis recorded MS-MS spectra of the peptides of interest. This brings us back to a key point made earlier in this chapter: coverage. To maximize the effectiveness of Sequest- and SALSA-based approaches to mapping protein modifications, we must obtain MS-MS spectra on as many of the peptides in the mixture as possible. This is why optimum protein digestion, peptide separation, and instrument sensitivity are critical to the task of protein modification mapping.

14.6. Integrating Sequest and SALSA to Map Protein Modifications

When used individually, both Sequest and SALSA have serious limitations for mapping protein modifications. Consider a realistic situation where we have obtained MS-MS spectra on a large number of peptides, both modified and unmodified, from a sample containing many different proteins. Sequest would detect predictable modifications on known amino acids (e.g., phosphoserine). However, Sequest generally would fail to detect modified forms when the nature and amino acid target of the modification are unanticipated. In this case, Sequest would attempt to correlate the spectrum of the modified peptide with a database of unmodified sequences. This would result in failure of Sequest to correctly match the spectrum to a correct amino acid sequence.

Analysis of the same data with SALSA would present a different problem. We could attempt to look for MS-MS spectra that displayed certain predictable characteristics, such as a neutral loss of phosphoric acid from phosphoserine and phosphothreonine. However, we again would fail to detect unanticipated modifications, or modifications that did not yield prominent losses or product ions, such as phosphotyrosine. The most effective way to detect modified peptide MS-MS spectra with SALSA is by sequence motif searching, as described earlier and in Chapter 10. However, to do this, we must know what motifs to search for. We cannot do that unless we know what proteins are represented in the sample.

This is where it makes sense to use Sequest and SALSA together (**Fig. 6**). The general approach is as follows. An initial analysis of the data with Sequest would successfully correlate many of the MS-MS

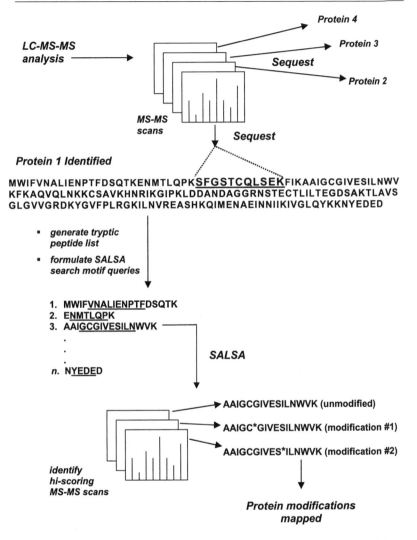

Fig. 6. Sequential application of LC-MS-MS, Sequest, and SALSA to identify protein components of a mixture and then to map modifications to the proteins.

spectra with database sequences. Even if some of the MS-MS spectra were of modified peptides and thus were not correctly identified by Sequest, other unmodified peptides from those same proteins would be identified. This initial Sequest search thus generates a list of proteins represented in the sample (e.g., Proteins 1, 2, 3, and 4 in **Fig. 6**).

Next, we perform SALSA searches for the sequence motifs represented by peptides from those proteins. These sequence motif searches identify not only the MS-MS spectra of the unmodified peptides (which probably were already identified by Sequest). The motif searches also identify MS-MS scans that have ion-series homology to the unmodified peptide spectra, yet have differences in the peptide masses and absolute m/z values of the product ions. These spectra correspond to the modified peptides. Inspection of these spectra will then allow deduction of the mass and sequence location of each modification. This combined Sequest/SALSA strategy is the most thorough way to identify and map modification on proteins.

Suggested Reading

Gatlin, C. L., Eng, J. K., Cross, S. T., Detter, J. C., and Yates, J. R., III (2000) Automated identification of amino acid sequence variations in proteins by HPLC/microspray tandem mass spectrometry. *Anal. Chem.* **72,** 757–763.

Liebler, D. C., Hansen, B. T., Davey, S. W., Tiscareno, L., and Mason, D. E. (2001) Peptide sequence motif analysis of tandem ms data with the SALSA algorithm. *Anal. Chem.*, in press.

Neubauer, G. and Mann, M. (1999) Mapping of phosphorylation sites of gel-isolated proteins by nanoelectrospray tandem mass spectrometry: potentials and limitations. *Anal. Chem.* **71,** 235–242.

Zhou, H., Watts, J. D., and Aebersold, R. (2001) A systematic approach to the analysis of protein phosphorylation. *Nat. Biotechnol.* **19,** 375–378.

15 New Directions in Proteomics

15.1. Evolving Techniques, Emerging Technologies

When we ask ourselves what we care about most in analytical proteomics work, two things spring to mind: *sensitivity* and *throughput*. Sensitivity is important because proteomics demands analysis of proteins at their natural abundance. In many cases, this forces us to analyze proteins that are present at very low levels. Throughput is important because, to really analyze *proteomes* (as opposed to proteins), we must be able to perform many analyses as rapidly as possible. Not surprisingly, proteomics technology is evolving toward both improved sensitivity and improved throughput.

These improvements are owing to evolution in both *technologies* and *techniques*. In this context, "technologies" refers to those instruments or instrumental approaches that provide fundamental capabilities, such as MS instruments, sources, chromatographic instrumentation, and so on. "Techniques," on the other hand, are the procedures we use to get the most out of the available instrumentation. It is important to distinguish these two areas, because improvements in both will drive future progress in proteomics.

Most of the instrumentation described earlier in this book has been available for at least five years. ESI-LC-MS-MS instruments have been in laboratories since the early 1990s and have enjoyed widespread use since 1996. MALDI-TOF instruments have been in use throughout

From: *Introduction to Proteomics: Tools for the New Biology*
By: D. C. Liebler © Humana Press, Inc., Totowa, NJ

the same period and the new high-resolution TOF analyzers have become widely used over the past five years. The capabilities of MS instruments have improved dramatically over this time period. Indeed, a typical MALDI-TOF or LC-MS system is over an order of magnitude more sensitive than the same instrument sold five years ago. This reflects improvements in mass analyzer technology, ESI and MALDI source design, detector sensitivity, and system electronics.

Much of the improvement in sensitivity for proteomics analyses has come from improved techniques for sample preparation and introduction for both MALDI-TOF and ESI-LC-MS. More efficient protein extraction and digestions produce better yields of proteins and peptides from complex samples. Improved sample cleanup procedures remove contaminating detergents and salts that interfere with ionization and MS analysis. Newer low-flow and low dead-volume LC systems ensure more efficient delivery of small sample amounts to MS instruments, which often perform best in conditions of low flow (*see* below). Thus, the community of researchers doing proteomics work and analytical protein biochemistry continues to develop better techniques that provide better sensitivity and, in some cases, better throughput.

These changes will continue to make proteome analyses more sensitive and will fuel continued rapid growth of proteomics. Nevertheless, other emerging technologies will produce even more impressive improvements in our ability to analyze proteomes. Four areas of emerging technologies are highlighted in the following sections.

15.2. New MS Instruments

Instrumentation for MS analysis of peptides and proteins is evolving at an impressive rate. This evolution involves both techniques and technologies. Although the sensitivity of mass analyzers and detectors has improved significantly, additional improvements in sensitivity have come from new approaches to sample preparation and introduction. Most notable among these "front-end" innovations is the introduction of ultra-low flow sample inlet systems for ESI-LC-MS instruments. The term "nanospray" is most commonly used to describe these techniques, in which sample flows into the ESI source are in the range of 50–500 nanoliters per minute (as opposed to 50–500 microliters per minute with more commonly used narrow-bore columns). A reduced flow rate for sample introduction results in more efficient transfer of peptide ions from the solution to the mass analyzer. This allows MS-MS analyses to be done on samples in the high attomole to low femtomole range, which is about two orders of magnitude lower than can be done with higher flow systems. Nanospray may be done with fused silica capillaries that are packed with HPLC separation media and thus function both as LC column and electrospray needle. Alternatively, samples may be simply loaded into unpacked nanospray needles and the peptides in the needle then are directed into the MS without in-line separation. In the application of multidimensional chromatography to tandem LC-MS-MS analyses, Yates and colleagues use fused silica capillaries packed with both ion exchange and RP LC separation media (*see* Chapter 4). Nanospray sources have been in use by many proteomics laboratories for the past 2–3 years. However, more widespread use of this approach has been limited in the past by the relatively delicate nature of available nanospray sources, the difficulty in interfacing these sources with automation tools (e.g., autosamplers), and a general lack of robustness of the available instrumentation. The outstanding sensitivity advantage offered by nanospray has led to the recent introduction of more reliable, user friendly commercial nanospray sources and accessories. The increasingly widespread use of nanospray techniques suggests that this will become the default LC-MS-MS mode for proteomics analyses.

Among the newer, more powerful MS instruments mentioned at the end of Chapter 6 are the Q-TOF (quadrupole-time of flight) and FT (Fourier transform) mass analyzers. FT instruments offer the ultimate in mass resolution and have been used increasingly to analyze complex mixtures of peptides. Accurate, high-resolution measurements of the masses of peptides in a complex mixture can permit protein identification by a variant of the peptide mass fingerprinting approach discussed in Chapter 7. Known peptide masses, termed "accurate mass tags" in FT analyses, can be used as unique identifiers in some cases. In principle, the accurate mass tag approach to proteome analysis can be very powerful and comprehensive. Major limitations to wider use of FT instruments are their great expense and rather delicate nature.

Q-TOF MS instruments (most commonly equipped with ESI sources) are becoming very widely used in proteomics work. A key advantage of the Q-TOF over ion traps and triple quad instruments is high mass resolution provided by the TOF mass analyzer. This provides higher resolution and (with an appropriate calibration) high mass accuracy, which enables easier *de novo* sequence interpretation from peptide MS-MS data. High accuracy for precursor ion selection and product ion analysis greatly facilitates accurate identification of protein sequences from MS-MS spectra with database correlation algorithms (*see* Chapter 9). Q-TOF instruments also offer high sensitivity that equals or exceeds that of the best ion trap and MALDI-TOF instruments. A recent extension of Q-TOF technology is the recent coupling of this mass analyzer to a MALDI rather that ESI source. This hybrid couples the advantages of MALDI ionization with the ability to perform true MS-MS analyses. This is in contrast to most MALDI-TOF instruments, which cannot do true MS-MS (*see* Chapter 6). Application of new quadrupole designs has recently given rise to a new generation of triple quadrupole instruments that will rival Q-TOF mass analyzers for resolution, mass accuracy, and sensitivity.

In addition to these improvements or further developments of existing MS technologies, new tandem mass analyzers are emerging. Most interesting among these is the TOF-TOF mass analyzer, which is a tandem mass analyzer in which two different time of flight analyzers are used for high-resolution precursor selection and product ion detection. In contrast to MALDI-TOF instruments, which cannot perform true MS-MS experiments, the TOF-TOF analyzer offers the prospect of high-throughput, MALDI-based MS-MS with exceptional resolution for precursor and product ions in MS-MS.

Another noteworthy development is the application of MS as a "virtual imaging" approach to the analysis of protein distributions in cell and tissue samples. Recent work indicates that it is possible to blot tissue slices onto a polyethylene membrane, coat with a MALDI matrix, and then perform a series of MALDI analyses distributed over the surface of the blot. Alignment of an ordered series of MALDI laser "shots" and recording of the spectra allows spectral patterns of peptide and protein masses to be recorded over the entire blot surface. Representation of the data for any particular mass will then indicate the spatial distribution of the corresponding protein or peptide in the tissue slice. Further development of this technology and eventual integration with tandem mass analyzers offers a powerful new tool to integrate proteomics and imaging in biological samples.

15.3. Automation and Robotics

In describing the analytical proteomics techniques in this book, we have focused on fundamental aspects. For example, in the analysis of 2D gels, we may select a number of protein spots for MS analysis. This implies that we will cut out each spot, subject each of these samples to in-gel digestion and MS analysis of the resulting peptides, then analyze the data with appropriate software. Although this approach is workable, it is limited in throughput. Moreover, individual differences in sample quality arise through inevitable variability in manual sample processing. Of course, the answer to this problem is the automation of as many steps in the analytical process as possible. Indeed, this is being done to an increasing extent to enhance the speed and reliability of proteome analyses.

In the case of 2D gels, several companies sell software to facilitate automated imaging of the protein spots in gels. Spot selection for subsequent analysis can be automated to a significant degree with the aid of pattern recognition and comparison algorithms. This software then drives automated "spot cutters," which harvest gel pieces and transfer them to robotic apparatus for automated digestion and preparation for MS analysis. In many cases, these robots actually can transfer the prepared samples to MALDI targets or to autosampler vials for LC-MS analyses. The automation of the entire process greatly improves the overall speed of proteome analyses. The high reproducibility of digestion and other sample preparation steps by robots diminishes sample-to-sample variability that inevitably accompanies manual sample preparation. In addition, the software controlling these automated systems provides automated sample tracking and related aspects of quality control, which is crucial to high-throughput analyses.

Postanalysis automation facilitates the analysis of data. For example, automated processing of MS datafiles permits completely automated or semi-automated protein identification from the data as it is being collected. Of course, the task of reviewing and interpreting the results of these analyses will always be with us. However, the power of automation tools for sample preparation, analysis, and data mining and organization is essential to the large-scale analysis of proteomes.

15.4. Micro- and Nanoscale Instrumentation

An important emerging theme in virtually all areas of technology is miniaturization. Miniature-scale technology is particularly applicable to high-sensitivity analytical work, because it brings the scale of the analytical tools closer to that of the targets of our analyses: proteins and peptides in cells. A major inefficiency in most of the techniques described in this book is that we are attempting to analyze picomoles or femtomoles of peptides in columns, gels, and MS sources with micrometer to millimeter internal dimensions. This difference in scale is like rolling a handful of marbles down the street and trying to recover them all at the other end. Losses are inevitable due to the many surfaces and components that peptides may interact with. Indeed, multiple material transfer steps (pipetting, chromatography, elution from gels, etc.) all present opportunities for peptides to be lost.

The idea of applying micro- or nanoscale separations and instrumentation is an effort to minimize the scale difference between analytes and apparatus and to minimize inefficiencies in analyses. Thus, much attention has recently been given to the development of microfluidic devices for extracting, digesting, and otherwise preparing proteins and peptides for MS analysis. Volumes for sample application to such devices are in the picoliter to microliter range. Numerous prototype devices have been reported in the public literature and others are in proprietary commercial development. A common characteristic of many of these devices is their construction on silicon chips similar to those used for microcircuits. This facilitates incorporation of electronic controls and of detectors into the devices.

New microscale analytical sample preparation or separation devices often employ parallel designs to facilitate the simultaneous processing and analysis of a number of samples at the same time. This addresses another imperative of proteome analysis: high throughput. As noted in earlier chapters, proteomics as described in much of this book fails to meet the standards for highly parallel analyses established by microarrays. Highly parallel devices that can facilitate digestion, separations, and MS analyses of multiple samples can greatly increase the speed of proteome analyses. Finally, microscale MS sources are being developed to efficiently couple microscale peptide separation devices to mass analyzers. Ionization methods used in prototypes for such sources include both MALDI and ESI. The sensitivity advantage offered by microscale sources is similar to that offered by nanospray. These microscale ionization sources offer highly efficient translation of sample ions to the mass analyzer.

15.5. Protein Arrays

Certainly the ultimate proteomics match to DNA microarrays would be protein arrays. Unfortunately, there is a major intrinsic problem with this approach. The basis for oligonucleotide array technology is the hybridization of complementary sequences via Watson-Crick base pairing. Unfortunately, proteins do not hybridize to complementary sequences. Thus, the one-to-one correspondence between targets and probes that makes oligonucleotide microarrays work is unavailable to proteomics researchers. Nevertheless, protein analysis by selective interaction of proteins or peptides with an array of different recognition elements is in development in a number of laboratories.

There are a number of different possible recognition elements for proteins. These range from relatively nonselective to highly selective recognition molecules. The former include ion exchange media, which bind proteins or peptides on the basis of charge under specific solution conditions, and immobilized metal affinity ligands, which recognize some protein functional groups, such as phosphoserine, phosphothreonine, and phosphotyrosine residues. The latter include antibodies, which are directed against specific proteins. MAbs directed against specific protein-sequence epitopes display the greatest selectivity for their protein targets. Nucleic acid *aptamers* represent another highly selective recognition element for proteins or peptides. Aptamers arise from the fact that different oligonucleotide sequences for unique arrangements of hydrogen-bonding donors and acceptors in three dimensional space. Thus, different oligonucleotide sequences may specifically bind to specific protein or peptide structural motifs.

These and other various recognition elements have been employed in proteome analyses as a step to extract specific protein or peptides from complex mixtures. Indeed, this approach has been extensively developed by Ciphergen Biosystems (www.ciphergen.com), which offers a large variety of customized surface "chips" for protein capture prior to MALDI-TOF MS analysis. Thus, the use of a relatively nonspecific capture surface harvests diverse proteins, whereas a more specific surface chemistry (e.g., a MAb) may trap only a single protein and some of its variants. Although the MALDI-TOF analysis of the intact proteins does not offer definitive identification, the analysis of changing "patterns" of proteins captured can provide a basis for more in-depth investigation.

Another way that arrays of protein recognition elements will impact proteomics is as an *alternative* to MS analysis, rather than as a front-end to capture proteins for MS. For example, arrays containing many different antibodies may be used to capture a diverse collection of proteins to which the antibodies are targeted. Use of non-MS detection strategies (e.g., secondary antibody labeling with fluorescent tags) can provide a very sensitive, high-throughput screen for the presence of specific proteins. Of course, the success of this approach depends on the specificity and affinity of the antibodies for their protein targets, on the effect of the antibody-attachment chemistry on antibody efficiency, and on the stringency of conditions under which the antibodies bind their protein targets. Related approaches also are evolving. For example, highly specific aptamer arrays can be envisioned, as the technology for aptamer generation and characterization is improving. The development of a high-throughput means of generating aptamers directed against specific proteins, peptides, or their modified variants could enable the construction of printed ologonucleotide arrays that are used for large-scale proteome analyses.

Another aspect of array approaches for proteomics is that they may serve as tools for more than mining proteomes. Arrays of specific proteins provide the opportunity to perform highly parallel studies of protein-protein interactions and how these interactions are affected by drugs and other chemical or physical factors. In this way, arrays of proteins printed on glass slides or in multiwell plates could be used to study protein-protein or protein-drug interactions in well-defined environments. Subsequent analyses of members of complexes or of protein modifications on individual elements of the arrays could then be performed with the MS tools described earlier in this book.

Suggested Reading

Baldwin, M. A., Medzihradsky, K. F., Lock, C. M., Fisher, B., Settineri, T. A., and Burlingame, A. L. (2001) Matrix-assisted laser desorption/ionization coupled with quadrupole/orthogonal acceleration time-of-flight mass spectrometry for protein discovery, identification and structural analysis. *Anal. Chem.* **73**, 1707–1720.

Chaurand, P., Stoeckli, M., and Caprioli, R. M. (1999) Direct profiling of proteins in biological tissue sections by MALDI mass spectrometry. *Anal. Chem.* **71**, 5263–5270.

Conrads, T. P., Alving, K., Veenstra, T. D., Belov, M. E., Anderson, G. A., Anderson, D. J., et al. (2001) Quantitative proteome analysis of bacterial and mammalian proteomes using a combination of cysteine affinity tags and ^{15}N-metabolic labeling. *Anal. Chem.* **73**, 2132–2139.

Figeys, D. and Pinto, D. (2000) Lab-on-a-chip: a revolution in biological and medical sciences. *Anal. Chem.* **72**, 330A–335A.

Lopez, M. F. (2000) Better approaches to finding the needle in a haystack: optimizing proteome analysis through automation. *Electrophoresis* **21**, 1082–1093.

MacBeth, G. and Schreiber, S. (2001) Printing proteins as microarrays for high-throughput function determination. *Science* **289**, 1760–1763.

Medzihradsky, K. F., Campbell, J. M., Baldwin, M. A., Falick, A. M., Juhasz, P., Vestal, M. L., and Burlingame, A. L. (2000) The characteristics of peptide collision-induced dissociation using a high performance MALDI-TOF/TOF tandem mass spectrometer. *Anal. Chem.* **72**, 552–558.

Zhu, H., Biolgin, M., Bangham, R., Hall, D., Casamayor, A., Bertone, P., Lan, N., Jansen, R., Bidlingmaier, S., Houfek, T., Mitchell, T., Miller, P., Dean, R. A., Gerstein, M. and Snyder, M. (2001) Global analysis of protein activities using proteome chips. *Science* **293**, 2101–2105.

Index